Hear For Life:

Dr. Joe's Guide To Your Child's Hearing Loss

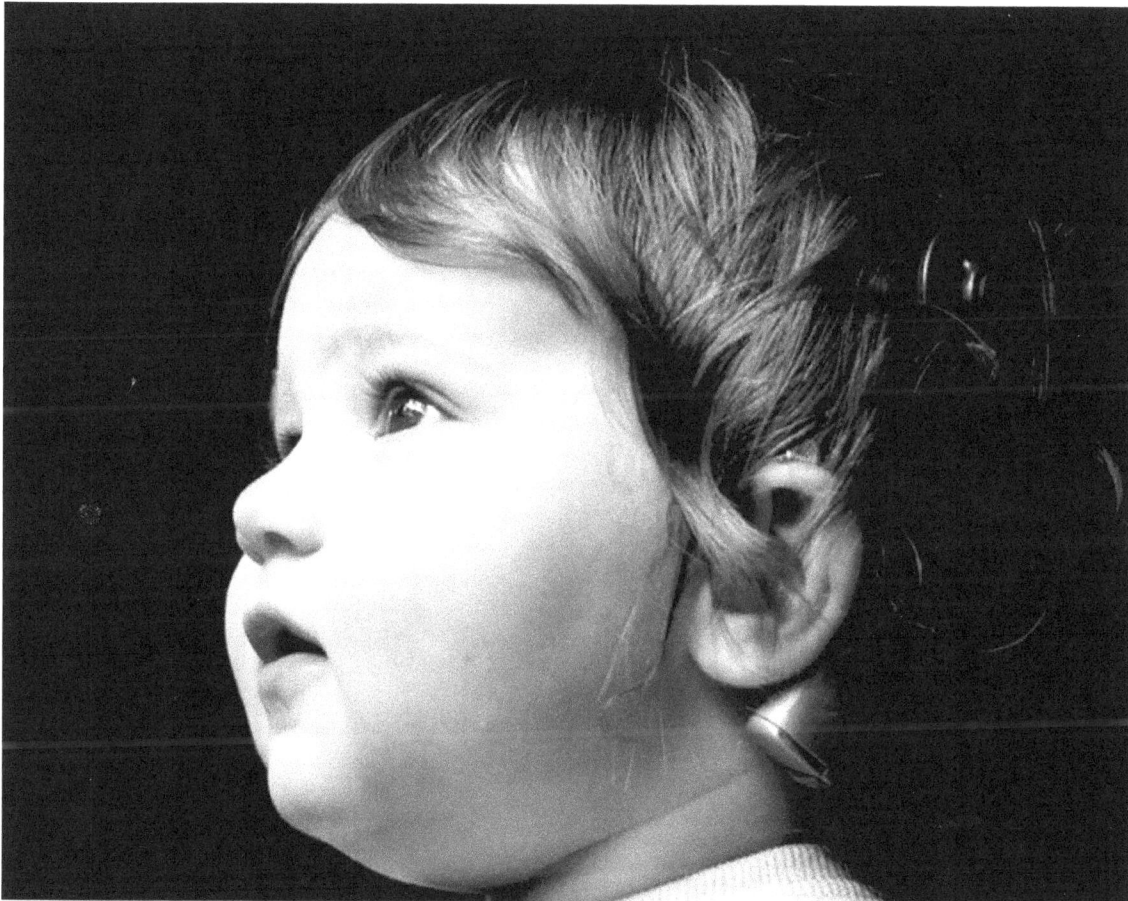

Joseph B. Roberson Jr., M.D.
Sheri Byrne-Haber, B.Sc., J.D.
Caitlin Roberson

LetThemHear.org

ISBN-10:0615774946
ISBN-13: 978-0-615-77494-7

ACKNOWLEDGMENT

Special thanks to the Prinz and Agnich families for lending us the images of their wonderful children.

Thanks to Allison Brower, Au.D., CCC-A for her diligent work on the manuscript of this book.

The herculean effort by Spencer Kirkland brought this book to completion!

Table of Contents

Foreword

Dr. Joseph B. Roberson, Jr.

You need to know that what you face is serious, because hearing impairment can have a severe impact on the life of the child who has it. You also need to understand that hearing impairment is treatable—beginning at birth. My purpose here is to give you, in a concentrated resource, the complete picture of how to get there. You will understand the tools and resources available for your use. I want you to have a glimpse of the end from the beginning.

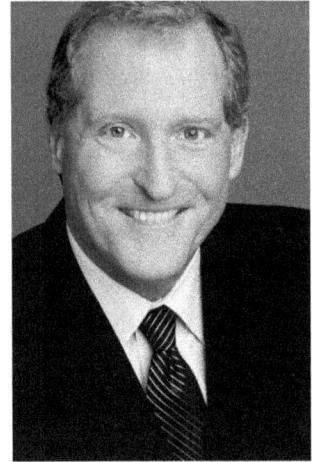

As a young boy, one of my favorite times of year was late spring, because my grandfather would let me accompany him as he prepared his fields for planting. He lived in another era, with limited economic resources, and turned the soil on his small farm using horse and plow. Mostly, I sat on the laboring horse in the hot sunshine holding onto the yoke and watching as we went back and forth over his field of many acres. Occasionally, I would help "man" the plow, as he placed his own strong hands over mine, steering the blade through the soft, warm earth. The long field where we labored was framed by a gravel road on one end, and on the other by a barbed-wire fence constructed with hickory fence posts every six feet or so.

This delightful man from the mountains of western North Carolina taught me that the best way to plow a straight furrow was to aim at a fence post, keeping it firmly in view throughout the entire length of the field. If I did not follow his advice, or if I lost sight of the objective, my furrow would curve this way and that, creating chaos in the field as I made my way from gravel road to fence line. What Granddad had the wisdom and presence of mind to teach me was that life is no different. Seeing the finish from the start will allow us to do our best without creating disorder and chaos on the way to the objective.

With this book, I want to help you make a strong start as you begin to see what your child can be—as you begin to see your child's end from the beginning. I want you to realize how important it is to educate yourself about hearing impairment, its effects, and the actions you can take to deal with it. My hope and prayer for you is that yours will be the steady and strong hand on the plow for your little one for as far as you are needed in the field of his or her life. Neither of us know what your offspring was made for, but we can work together to make sure the hearing, listening (they are different!), receptive and expressive language, and cognitive development your child can have are ready when they're needed.

Sheri Byrne-Haber

On August 25, 1991, I was packing my things in Rockyview Hospital in Calgary, Alberta. After a fairly difficult pregnancy, I had given birth to my second daughter the day before, and I was ready to go home. When I went to the head nurse to inquire about getting discharged, she said to me, "Don't you want to wait for the ENT to get here? It takes a while to get them out on Sundays."

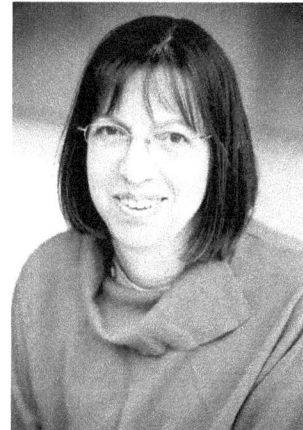

Little did I know that one single comment was my introduction to being the parent of a child with a significant congenital hearing impairment. Because my daughter had been born with two different-sized ears, the protocol in Canada was to automatically conduct an infant hearing examination. Today, infant hearing screening is mandated in the majority of the states in the United States. My daughter's chart had a "blue card" in it, meaning she had not passed the infant hearing screening examination and was referred for additional follow-up testing. At four months of age, she was diagnosed with a bilateral mixed hearing impairment due to branchiootorenal syndrome.

Sixteen years later, she is the poster child for how a child with a congenital hearing impairment can lead an absolutely normal life in a hearing world. She sings in the choir, speaks Mandarin, plays the flute and the guitar, and is making plans for college. The road to achieve that normalcy was not without bumps, and required significant family commitment as well as medical treatment and therapy, but it is a road that I am glad that we travelled, and one that I would like to share with everyone who finds themselves in the same situation that I did sixteen years ago. It is a road that, as the parent of a child with a hearing impairment, I urge all families to consider.

Author's Note

This book uses "People First" language in describing hearing impairment and people who have hearing impairment. The authors have deliberately chosen to consistently use the phrase "individuals with hearing impairment" because we believe it most accurately describes both the condition and the people with the condition. We believe that the terms "hard of hearing," "deaf," and "Deaf" are either not as accurate, or contain emotional connotations that this book does not intend to address.

When using the term "disability" to refer to a hearing impairment in this book, the authors are always referring to U.S. federal government statutes, which occasionally define hearing impairment as a "disability." Whether or not hearing impairment *is* a disability, or whether an individual with a hearing impairment thinks of himself or herself as disabled because of the hearing impairment, is not a question the authors intend to address in this book.

Chapter 1
Earliest Days

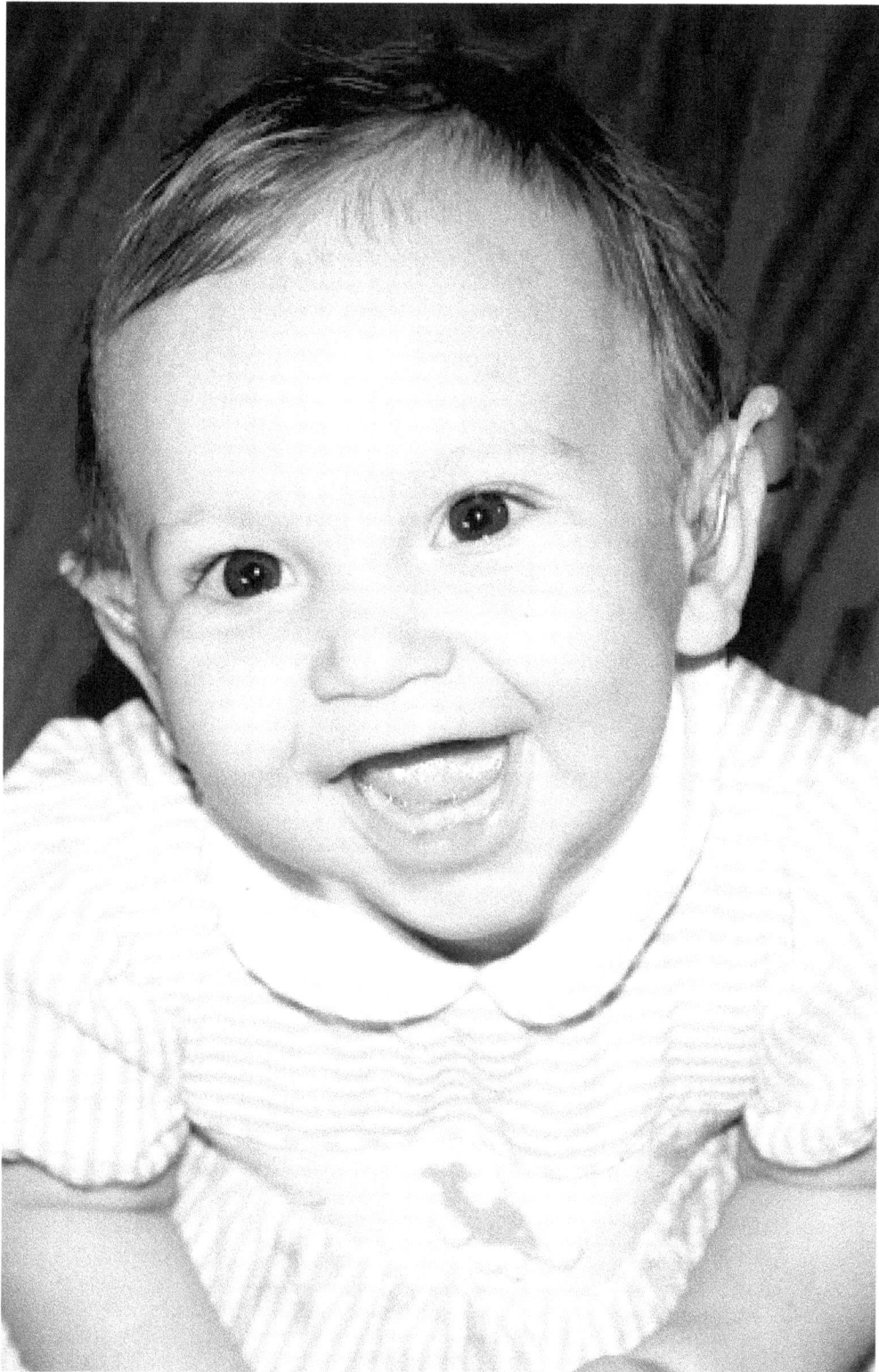

Introduction

If you have picked up this book, it is likely that your child or someone you know was recently diagnosed with hearing loss. Without a doubt, what you face is serious. However, there is good news: Hearing loss is treatable, and treatment may start at birth. If you want your child to hear and speak and live in a hearing world, then this book is for you.

Chances are you're experiencing an array of emotions at this moment: perhaps sadness, maybe anger, even guilt. Perhaps you feel intimidated and overwhelmed. This is a normal reaction that all parents have. It is disappointing beyond words to face any type of difficulty out of the blue, and hearing impairment is no exception.

We understand. Talk about it. Cry about it. Find others who have walked this road before you and talk about it with them. They have also talked and cried about it; of that we have no doubt. Express your feelings to your hearing health provider. Talk about it with the whole family, including extended family members. Some people find that enlisting a counselor helps. Lend this book to people whose opinions matter to you if they need the knowledge you are about to get. Each person and family has a unique way of coming to grips with their own situation.

If you are facing this as a couple, it is essential to be sensitive to your mate. You may not be on the same page with your significant other in either the grieving process or the process of creating a plan for your child's future. Different people will have different issues and will go through their feelings at different rates. With loving patience and understanding as a foundation, try hard to get on the same page. Your child needs you there.

As parents, you need to become the ultimate decision makers for your child, so that you can find the best resolution and create an effective plan for reaching it. The good news is that you have come to the right place. Relying on this book and hearing health professionals, you will begin to educate yourself to make choices for your family. Only you, as a parent, know what is right for your child and your family. You have to be in control of the overall care group you choose for your child. Think of yourself as the coach of a team—a team that you put together, and whose activities you direct. Each player has a defined role, with you acting as the overall coordinator. In a later chapter, we will describe team members and their individual positions. You will need to investigate what players are available in your area and make your draft choices.

It takes most parents years to achieve the knowledge base they need to overcome the effects of hearing loss in their children's lives. We've written this book to make the process easier for you. Think of it as your one-stop resource.

There is a lot of information here, so don't be overwhelmed. We've arranged the information chronologically in bite-size chunks—from birth to school and beyond—so that you can use what you need now, and refer back to it later on. Our goal is to give you a glimpse of the end from the beginning.

You will never regret the time, effort, and financial resources you put into this process. Done right, the payoff is something you will observe for the remainder of your life and your child's life. You can do it, Coach! And we will show you how.

Here's your first assignment: Find out if a hearing impairment is present, what caused it, and what you are going to do about it. Let's begin.

Hearing impairment is the most common birth defect in the world, affecting three to four infants per 1,000 births. Hearing impairment can also be acquired through infection, tumor, and adverse reaction to medication, trauma, or noise. The frequency of hearing impairment increases with age, making it the most common medical condition in humans. Today, more than 22 million Americans have some form of hearing impairment, and 1 in 400 Americans is profoundly hearing impaired. If left untreated, hearing impairment is a very expensive medical condition, and it can be socially and psychologically damaging. When hearing loss in infants is not identified, or when they do not receive early intervention services, it can cost an average of $420,000 per child in special education services. The lifetime cost to society can top $1 million per individual.

Hearing impairment during the first years of life can result in widespread, severe, lifelong, and irreversible limitations in speech and language development. If parents want their children to hear and communicate orally, they must pursue early, aggressive treatment, including the use of hearing devices or cochlear implants, combined with customized therapy and training modalities. Therapy can prevent the disastrous effect of hearing impairment on infant language development, allowing instead for normal development and achievement.

The ability to provide successful medical treatment for hearing-impaired individuals has changed drastically during the past thirty years. Up until the 1980s, parents who wanted their children with severe to profound hearing impairments to speak, rather than use sign language, as their primary mode of communication frequently had no options other than analog hearing aids and intensive speech therapy. Even with the best treatment possible, up until the 1980s, the results were often less than what the parents had hoped for.

In 1980, the U.S. Food and Drug Administration approved the first cochlear implant for use in adults. In 1986, they were approved for children. These initial cochlear implants had one electrode. Today, current implants use twenty-four electrodes, plus powerful speech processors that are worn either on the body or behind the ear. The speech processors allow for software upgrades designed to improve the processing of the electrode implanted inside the cochlea without additional surgery. Similarly, hearing technology has improved and is now available in digital form. Cochlear implants are used with the most severe hearing loss, while hearing aids are used with less severe hearing loss. Many more children use hearing aids than cochlear implants.

When cochlear implants were first approved for children, the average age at which a child was first identified with hearing loss was three years of age. The delay in identification was due to the fact that in the 1980s, only children who were considered to be at high risk for hearing impairment received infant hearing screenings. More than 94 percent of children born with hearing loss are born to parents with normal hearing. As a result, these children are not considered high-risk and did not receive a hearing screening. Often, the child's hearing loss went undetected until the child was approximately two to three years old and had failed to develop normal speech and language skills.

When hearing impairment in infants goes undetected, there are significant and negative effects on speech, language, social, and emotional development, as well as academic achievement. A 1996 Gallaudet Research Institute in-depth study of reading skills in deaf and hard-of-hearing high school seniors revealed that their average reading level was the same as that of fourth-grade students with normal hearing—an astounding seven- to eight-year delay.

Major advancements have been made in cochlear implant technology and infant hearing screening in the past decade. As a result, the medical community has been able to lessen the effects of late identification of hearing impairment in infants. The majority of states now have a law in place making newborn hearing screening mandatory.[3][1] This has significantly leveled the playing field for profoundly hearing-impaired infants. For example, in Colorado, the average age of identification of hearing-impaired children has decreased from twenty-four to thirty months of

---

[1] [3] National Center for Hearing Assessment and Management (NCHAM) on National Institutes of Health (NIH) Consensus Development Conference on Early Identification of Hearing Loss (1993) http://www.infanthearing.org/screening/index.html

age to two months of age.[4][2] This aggressive movement toward earlier identification has provided the medical community with an important opportunity to significantly diminish the negative and pervasive developmental impact of hearing impairment through earlier medical and therapeutic intervention.

For the two-thirds of children with congenital hearing impairment who can benefit from hearing aids, digital technology represents a significant advance in amplification. Directional microphones and software programs, which boost the understandability of speech while suppressing the amplification of background noise, have also provided a substantial improvement to the hearing aid user.

To be sure, hearing impairment can produce devastating effects on speech, language, and school performance, among other problems. If not properly treated, or if treated too late, hearing impairment will limit options for your child's life. With quick, effective, and appropriate treatment, the majority of children can lead lives in a hearing and speaking world alongside their normally hearing peers. Many children and adults with hearing impairments function normally and are not limited in any way by their hearing impairment. Using the knowledge and guidelines detailed in this book, you can achieve the best outcomes for your child.

Some parents choose not to restore hearing to their hearing-impaired children, accepting the effects that the hearing impairment will have on their children's language development, school setting, and life choices. These children become part of the Deaf culture, and usually rely on sign language as their primary mode of communication. These children can also lead

---

[2] [4] http://www.colorado.edu/slhs/mdnc/research/publications/itano.html

wonderfully productive and fulfilling lives.

Newly Diagnosed Hearing Loss

It is extremely important to act quickly once the diagnosis of hearing impairment is made or suspected in your child. The human hearing system develops rapidly from before birth and during the first few years of life. If critical periods of development are missed, no amount of intervention can correct those losses. The age at which the treatment began is the single most important factor in predicting successful treatment of congenital hearing impairment in children. If you are one of the 94 percent of families who are hearing parents of a child suspected to have a hearing impairment, you are currently being bombarded with decisions you know little or nothing about. The infant hearing screening is completed with an automated machine and is often performed by personnel or volunteers of the hospital. Although they may know how to operate the equipment, they may not have any knowledge or experience about how to advise parents whose children do not pass the screening.

The infant hearing screening is extremely simple and is designed to identify children with normal hearing. Those children whose test results do not meet the definition of normal hearing are referred for further testing. Further testing by an experienced physician-audiologist team is necessary to determine whether your child has a hearing impairment. In some cases, the abnormal screening test can be a false alarm, and children who are referred may actually have normal hearing. For example, fluid or debris in the ear canal after birth can create a temporary hearing impairment that results in a referral. However, once the fluid or debris is gone, the child's hearing is in fact normal.

Unfortunately, other children can pass infant hearing screening examinations initially because they have a progressive hearing impairment. A progressive hearing impairment is a type of hearing loss that develops over time and has not yet fully evolved at birth. Therefore, the infant hearing screening is not foolproof, but is just one tool that is used to help identify children who may need a more in-depth diagnostic evaluation of their hearing systems.

If a hearing impairment is indeed present, it needs to be defined and characterized. True deafness—the inability to hear any sound at any level of loudness—is present in less than 3 percent of children with hearing impairment. In all other cases, some level of hearing remains. The amount of hearing impairment can vary widely both in intensity (decibel level) and pitch (frequency). To know what treatment is needed for your child, the exact levels of how many decibels are lost and at which frequencies must be determined.

Some forms of hearing impairment are progressive. A child can pass an infant hearing screening and then develop hearing impairment over time. In other situations, they can be referred from infant hearing screening and initially be diagnosed with a mild or moderate hearing impairment that later gets worse over time. In some cases, a child may not have received an infant hearing screening and is later suspected of having a hearing impairment because of behavior in certain listening situations and/or lack of proper language development. Evaluation by a competent professional is very important and will bring clarity to the situation.

For children without infant hearing screening, the average age of identification of hearing impairment has not changed in many years and is generally well over eighteen months. Loss of these early months of development can have negative effects on the child, and in some circumstances can prevent the best possible speech and language development.

If your child is referred from an infant hearing screening examination, your first task is to schedule a follow-up exam and testing with a hearing health care provider. Hearing testing can be accurately performed from birth onward by clinics with modern techniques, training, and equipment. Sometimes, parents are told hearing testing cannot be accurately performed until the child is older. If you hear this inaccurate statement, keep looking for a provider with the experience, up-to-date knowledge, and ability to test your child accurately. Accurate test results are extremely important, regardless of what communications route you end up choosing for your child. Selecting a follow-up testing facility is a very important decision—you may be choosing a group with which you will partner to treat your child's hearing impairment for many years—so asking around to find out who is the best in your area is well worth the effort.

Early Intervention Needed

The brain needs normal sound delivered to it in the first months and years of life to develop normal sound pathways in the brain. If sound is not present during these periods, the brain's ability to develop these sound pathways is permanently lost. These periods of development are present in many human systems and are part of how we are made. The medical term for this is a "critical period of development."

For example, if a child is ten years old and has never had sound input at any time, then learning to talk normally is simply not possible, regardless of how much intervention the child receives. Language develops very early in life, and by ten years of age, the critical period of development is over and the brain cannot recover. The child cannot learn to talk beyond that point even if normal hearing is restored and the child begins intense speech training therapy. In fact, most of the development of the auditory-verbal system has occurred by five years of age.

For this reason, patients who receive treatment during their first five years of life develop both expressive (speaking) and receptive (listening) language more quickly and more fully. *The earlier they receive the intervention, the better.* Children begin to respond to sound at twenty weeks of pregnancy. Therefore, a child who is born with a congenital hearing impairment is already four to five months behind in "hearing age" compared to children with normal hearing.

One leading report stated:

> The children who underwent cochlear implantation at younger than 12 mo. of age achieved mean rates of receptive (1.12) and expressive (1.01) language growth that were ***comparable to their normally hearing peers*** and were significantly greater than the rates achieved by children who underwent implantation between 12 and 24 mo. of age.[5][3]

Another leading study concluded:

> [T]he onset of babbling takes place and seems to be triggered by the cochlear implant. It took a median of 1 month of auditory exposure to start babbling regardless of the age of implantation. Because babbling in normally hearing children starts at a mean age of 8 months, only very early cochlear implantation is able to keep the infants within the normal age range. The impact of age of implantation was very clear: the earlier the implantation, the earlier the onset of babbling and good auditory performance. Even in the 5-20 months age group, the earlier the implantation, the better the results appeared to be in line with those of normally hearing children.[6][4]

In many situations, five-year-old children with hearing impairment who began appropriate treatment and therapy before their first birthday show no differences from children with normal hearing in their speech and language development. Children with congenital hearing impairments who do not receive treatment until three years of age, in contrast, are on average significantly behind the speech and language development of children their age with normal

---

[3] [5] Dettman, S.J., Pinder, D., Briggs, R.J., Dowell, R.C., and Leigh, J.R. "Communication Development in Children Who Receive the Cochlear Implant Younger Than 12 Months: Risks Versus Benefits." *Ear Hear* 28 (2 Suppl) (Apr. 2007): 11S-18S.

[4] [6] Schauwers, K., Gillis, S., Daemers, K., De Beukelaer, C., Govaerts, P.J. "Cochlear Implantation Between 5 and 20 Months of Age: The Onset of Babbling and the Audiologic Outcome." *Otol Neuroto.* 25 (3) (May 2005): 263-70.

hearing. With appropriate intervention, many of these children can catch up to their peers, but even then, they might not be reaching their full potential. Said another way, development time that is lost before intervention occurs can never be fully regained. If you and your child are fortunate enough to have discovered the hearing impairment early, you are in a position to make a large difference in the long-term effects it will have on your child.

In summary, define your child's hearing impairment immediately, and start treatment as soon as possible. Now that you know how important it is to address this issue, let's give you the knowledge you'll need to get it done.

The Anatomy of the Ear

The ear is divided into three sections, each responsible for a different part of hearing: the inner ear, middle ear, and outer ear.

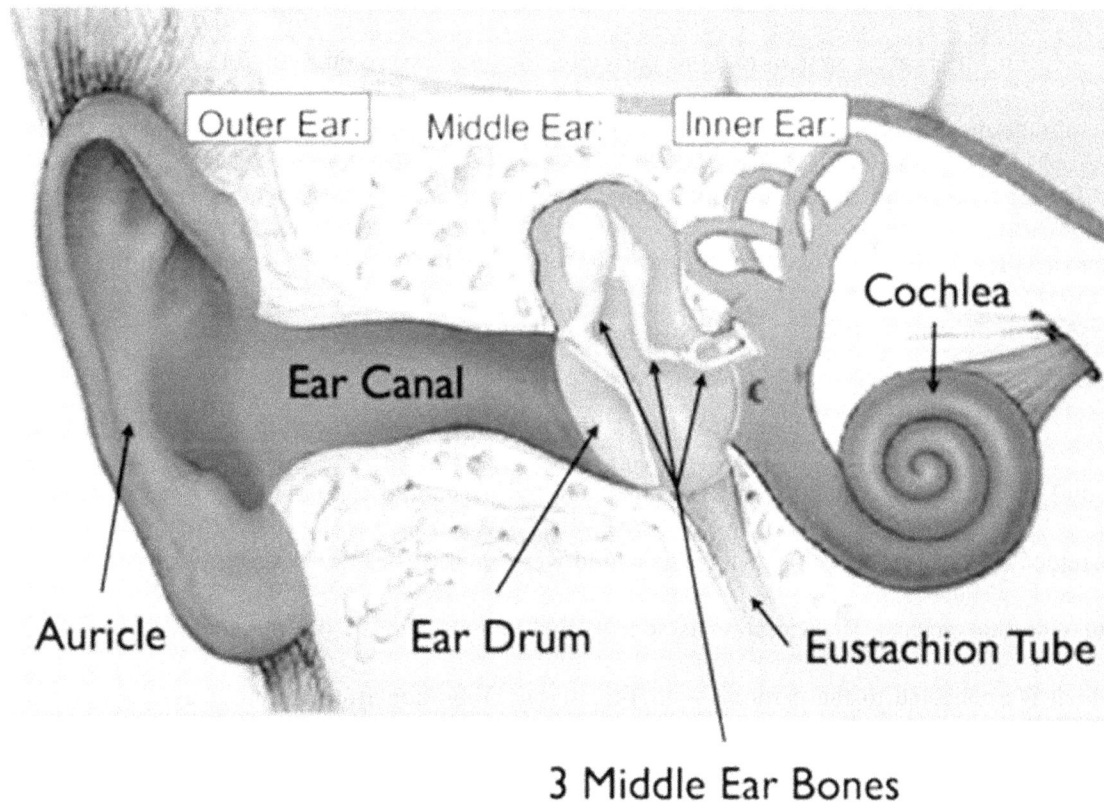

Outer Ear: Middle Ear: Inner Ear:

Cochlea

Ear Canal

Auricle   Ear Drum   Eustachion Tube

3 Middle Ear Bones

How Does Hearing Work?

Sound is a complex vibration transmitted through the air. Obviously, we cannot see the energy waves, but they can be demonstrated by imagining a stone thrown into a pond. As the stone breaks the surface of the water, a wave goes out in all directions until it strikes an object. Sound operates in a similar fashion. When the stone strikes the water, sound is generated. The sound wave travels in all directions away from the sound source.

The purpose of the hearing system is to take this vibrational energy, process it, and change it into electrical energy for the brain to process as nerve impulses. The outer ear (or pinna), the ear canal (or external auditory canal), the eardrum (or tympanic membrane), and the middle ear bones (or ossicles) work together to deliver the vibrations of sound to the fluid-filled inner ear, or cochlea.

For the hearing system to work correctly, the air pressure on both sides of the tympanic membrane must be the same. The eustachian tube opens and closes at different times to achieve pressure equalization. An example of normal opening of the eustachian tube occurs when you hear a soft sound when swallowing, or when your ear "pops" when changing altitude in an airplane or on a mountain.

Let's think of the stone thrown into the pond again. The pressure wave created by the sound enters the ear canal, where it is enhanced by the natural tone of the ear canal, which is designed to focus on speech signals. The sound wave then strikes the eardrum, where an in-and-out vibration occurs. The vibration is sent to the malleus, one of the three middle ear bones, which is connected to the eardrum with firm tissue. Vibration from the malleus is sent to the remainder of the ossicular chain: first the incus and then the stapes. The base of the stapes comes in contact with the fluid of the inner ear. A flexible ligament around the stapes allows it to move in and out, causing a vibration that moves into the snail-shaped cochlea.

The cochlea is tonotopic, meaning pertaining to the spatial arrangement of where sound is perceived. Think of the cochlea as a chamber measuring about an inch in length that is rolled up into a snail shell shape. Imagine the snail shell straightened out. Different pitches of sound are heard at different places along the length of the structure, much like the keys of a piano. The high-pitched sounds are heard closer to the right-hand end of the unrolled snail shell (towards the stapes), and the lower-pitched sounds are heard at the left-hand side of the unrolled snail shell (the tip of the chamber).

The inner ear is an extremely delicate system of membranes and nerve receptor cells. Nerve receptor cells anchored to the membranes turn the mechanical vibration delivered to the inner ear fluid into electrical energy. Small projections that look like hairs (thus giving these cells their names, *hair cells,* although they have nothing to do with human hair) bend and cause an electrical pulse to be transmitted along nerve endings.

Think of these hair cells as thin blades of grass on the bottom of a pond. As the current moves, as the grass sways to and fro, the roots of each blade of grass fire an electrical impulse. Each hair cell (or blade of grass) makes a connection called a synapse with hearing nerve cells further up the hearing pathway called spiral ganglion cells. The spiral ganglion cells send connections to the brain. Thousands of spiral ganglion cells located in the center of the turns of the cochlea send small fibers, called axons, to the brain. The collection of axons of the spiral ganglion cells form the hearing or auditory nerve. The auditory nerve connects, or synapses, with the cochlear nucleus—the next collection of nerve cells in the hearing chain, located in the area of the central nervous system between the spinal cord and the part of the brain called the brainstem. From the cochlear nucleus, axons continue on to both sides of the brain as they carry the sound to higher centers, where we then hear the sound.

The complete hearing system is very small. For example, the entire inner ear only has a few drops of fluid in it. In addition to hearing, the single cavity of the inner ear also contains the balance system. Surgeons need microscopes to perform surgery.

In general, as the hearing signal moves from its origin in the cochlea to where we perceive it in the brain, it becomes more organized. Processing, or organization, of the signal occurs at each level of the auditory system. In its simplest form, however, the inner ear is responsible for detecting sound and delivering a clear signal to the brain. The brain is responsible for selecting the portion of the signal we want to listen to.

A perfectly functioning inner ear will deliver a signal to the brain like a very expensive stereo system. All the notes are clear, crisp, and understandable, as well as enjoyable. A dysfunctional inner ear will deliver a sound more like an AM radio station, full of static or worse. Sometimes the sound is so bad, it sounds like a radio station that is too far away or slightly out of tune. Some understandable information is coming through, and if you concentrate very hard, you may be able to understand some of the information. In this situation, hearing takes a lot of effort, and the brain has to work to help understand what is being said.

In still other situations, virtually no sound is coming from the inner ear. Clearly, it is much more difficult, if not impossible, for normal speech and language to develop if the inner ear is not sending a clear sound to the brain. A child has to hear words clearly before he or she can say them clearly. If the speech signal is garbled or unclear, as in our radio example, the speech produced will be garbled or unclear. Different types of hearing impairment affect the speech signal differently.

In some cases, the inner ear is relaying a clear signal, but the brain's ability to select the important parts of the signal delivered to it can be impaired. Professionals call this a central auditory processing disorder, or CAPD.

Imagine yourself in a busy restaurant. Your inner ear is doing a good job and is changing the vibrational signals entering your ear canal into electrical impulses. The brain is getting a clear idea of all the sound in your environment: music in the background, clinking of glasses and forks on plates, chairs scooting, other conversations at tables near you, the crackling fire of the open grill behind the counter, the laughter of people across the room, the conversation of the person across the table. The brain focuses on the conversation coming from your dinner partner while ignoring the other sounds, allowing you to hear what is being said. However, as the background noise gets louder and louder, it eventually reaches a level at which even a perfectly functioning inner ear and brain can't pick out the sound you want to hear.

As hearing impairment worsens, this "line of understanding" shifts. This concept is called the signal-to-noise ratio. As background noise approaches or even exceeds the volume of the speech (i.e. signal) you want to hear, it becomes much harder to pick out the speech from the noise. All patients with hearing impairment have difficulty with background noise. Keep in mind that classrooms are among the noisiest environments possible. Therefore, producing the best sound possible from the ear and improving the signal-to-noise ratio of your child's classroom environment are both especially important.

For an interactive and animated description of how hearing works, visit the Let Them Hear Foundation website at http://www.letthemhear.org/hearing/implants.php# and click on "View the animations to learn about hearing."

How Is Hearing Impairment in Children Identified?

Ninety-four percent of children with hearing impairments are born to families with no significant history of hearing impairment. Even as recently as fifteen years ago, unless a child had one or more significant risk factors, hearing impairment frequently went unidentified until age three. At that age, it is clear that children with hearing impairments are failing to meet language development milestones. Today, the advent of newborn hearing screening means that a significant number of children, even those with zero risk factors, are being identified as hearing-impaired before even leaving the nursery to go home the first time.

After technology improvements, the single greatest positive impact on the treatment of hearing impairment has come from earlier identification of hearing impairment in infants as a result of state-based infant hearing screening programs (IHSPs).

As of 2005, 69 percent of all infants born in the United States were screened for hearing impairment before they left the newborn nursery. This has helped to lower the age of treatment. In states that are extremely aggressive with family follow-up, the average age at which a child receives amplification has been reduced from thirty-six months to ten months. However, this is not the case everywhere. In the United States as a whole, far too many facilities and families are failing to follow up with children who have been identified as potentially hearing-impaired.

Of those infants who were identified to have possible hearing impairment, just over half (56 percent) received the additional testing they needed by three months of age. Moreover, only 53 percent of the children who did receive follow-up testing and were officially diagnosed with a hearing impairment were enrolled in early intervention programs by six months of age. Combining these factors, the results are staggering. Only 20 percent of hearing-impaired infants born in the United States are being properly assessed and followed by six months of age. Unfortunately, the remaining 80 percent of children are not identified as hearing-impaired until much later.

What Causes Hearing Impairment?

Non-Genetic Congenital Sources of Hearing Impairment

Hearing impairment has many sources, including numerous genetic sources, non-genetic congenital sources (meaning those that are present at birth), and noncongenital sources. The following congenital conditions are highly linked to hearing impairment:

- Extreme prematurity has a high rate of association with hearing impairment due to auditory neuropathy, as well as several of the issues below.

- Non-premature twins are more likely to have hearing impairment when the weight difference between the twins is more than one pound, or when twin-to-twin transfusion syndrome is present.

- Ototoxic drug exposure is linked to hearing impairment. Children who are premature or who have significant medical events immediately after their birth may be given drugs that save their lives at the cost of their hearing. Aminoglycoside antibiotics such as Gentamycin or diuretics such as Lasix have been shown to cause hearing impairment in infants.

- Hyperbilirubinemia is the presence of an excess amount of bilirubin, which is linked to a temporary liver condition known as jaundice. Jaundice is most typically known for causing babies to have a yellowish color to their skin, especially noticeable in the whites of their eyes. High levels of bilirubin are generally initially treated with fluorescent light therapy (called bili-lights). However, if the bilirubin levels do not respond to this therapy or if the levels are extremely high, the baby may require a blood transfusion known as an "exchange." Levels of bilirubin high enough to require blood transfer exchanges have been linked to hearing impairment.

• Cytomegalovirus (CMV) is an infection that many people have had and don't know it. If contracted by the mother during pregnancy, it can be associated with hearing impairment.

• Although it has not been a significant issue in developed countries since the late 1960s to early 1970s, rubella infection (also known as German measles) during pregnancy used to be a significant cause of congenital hearing impairment. This can still be an issue when women have not received vaccines either by choice, because of allergies, or because they are living in a country where vaccines are either unavailable or not mandated by law.

• Hypoxia is caused by a lack of oxygen. The two most common causes of hypoxia for infants are having the umbilical cord wrapped around the neck during delivery or having an umbilical cord with fewer than the normal number of blood vessels present in it.

• Cochlear malformations can cause hearing impairment. While occasionally genetic, cochlear malformations are frequently isolated, meaning they are not part of a syndrome and there is no family history of cochlear malformations.

Acquired Hearing Impairment

Other forms of hearing impairment are not congenital but "acquired" and occur later in childhood. Several types of infections, which can develop any time after birth, can cause significant and sometimes permanent hearing impairment. The most common is chronic otitis media. However, viral infections can cause single-sided deafness (deafness of one ear only). Meningitis, both bacterial and viral, is also associated with acquired hearing impairment.

A cholesteatoma is a growth of skin cells occurring behind the eardrum that causes damage to the eardrum and the middle ear bones and can lead to more serious problems, including chronic ear infections, permanent hearing impairment, and dizziness. Cholesteatomas are most frequently described as benign (noncancerous) cysts in the middle ear.

Cholesteatomas may be acquired or congenital. The most common type of cholesteatoma is acquired, meaning that the cholesteatoma grows over time in a previously healthy ear. In these cases, the problem starts with a hole in the eardrum, known as an eardrum perforation. Eardrum perforations can result from ear infections, trauma, or a long-term difficulty in being able to equalize or "pop" the ears when changing altitudes or when suffering from congestion. After the hole is created, the opportunity exists for healthy skin cells to move from the ear canal and begin growing behind the eardrum.

Some individuals have congenital cholesteatomas, meaning they are born with the cholesteatoma growth already existing behind an intact eardrum. These cholesteatomas frequently go unnoticed for a long time, as they may be difficult to see behind the eardrum. It is thought that congenital cholesteatomas arise from cells that get misdirected during fetal development. Instead of forming cells that normally occur in the middle ear, they form skin cells instead.

Cholesteatoma treatment, at a minimum, requires surgery to remove the growth. Antibiotics can decrease associated infections, but there is no medication that will cure cholesteatomas. Surgery results in a safe, healthy ear, free of disease, and can also result in improvements in hearing lost due to the cholesteatoma. The procedure most commonly used to remove a cholesteatoma growth is called a tympanomastoidectomy. This outpatient surgery is completed in one and a half to two hours, with the patient going home the same day.

For patients with moderate to large cholesteatomas, a two-stage series of surgeries is recommended. The first procedure is completed to remove the cholesteatoma growth and clean up any associated chronic infections. The second surgery, completed six to nine months after the first, is a reexamination to make certain that no skin cells have regrown. During the second surgery, damaged middle ear bones (ossicles) can be repaired, or if too damaged to repair, they can be replaced with titanium prosthetics.

Other sources of acquired hearing impairment can include excessive exposure to noise, Ménière's disease, autoimmune inner ear disease, and tumors, including acoustic neuroma, glomus, and cholesterol granuloma. Most of these conditions are associated with adult-onset hearing impairment. Only a handful of children have ever been conclusively diagnosed with any of these conditions.

Key Takeaways

1. Hearing impairment is the most common birth defect in the world, affecting three to four infants per 1,000 births. It can be congenital (present at birth) or acquired (developing later in life).

2. Law now mandates newborn hearing screening in the majority of states.

3. If hearing impairment goes unnoticed or untreated, it can result in significant and negative effects on speech, language, social, and emotional development, as well as academic achievement.

4. Time is of the essence. It is imperative to work quickly to determine if your child has a hearing impairment, and if so, to begin effective and appropriate treatment as soon as possible.

5. The earlier a child begins treatment and intervention, the better outcomes in development will be seen.

6. Accurate diagnosis of the type and level of hearing impairment is extremely important.

7. Do your homework before choosing a physician-audiologist team. If your child is diagnosed with hearing loss, you may be working with this group for many years to come.

8. Digital hearing aids are used to treat less severe hearing loss, while cochlear implants are used with the most severe hearing loss. Many more children use hearing aids than cochlear implants.

9. The ear is composed of three sections: the outer ear, the middle ear, and the inner ear. All parts work together to deliver sound vibrations to the brain. Remember the stone-thrown-into-a-pond analogy.

Chapter 2

Immediate Next Steps

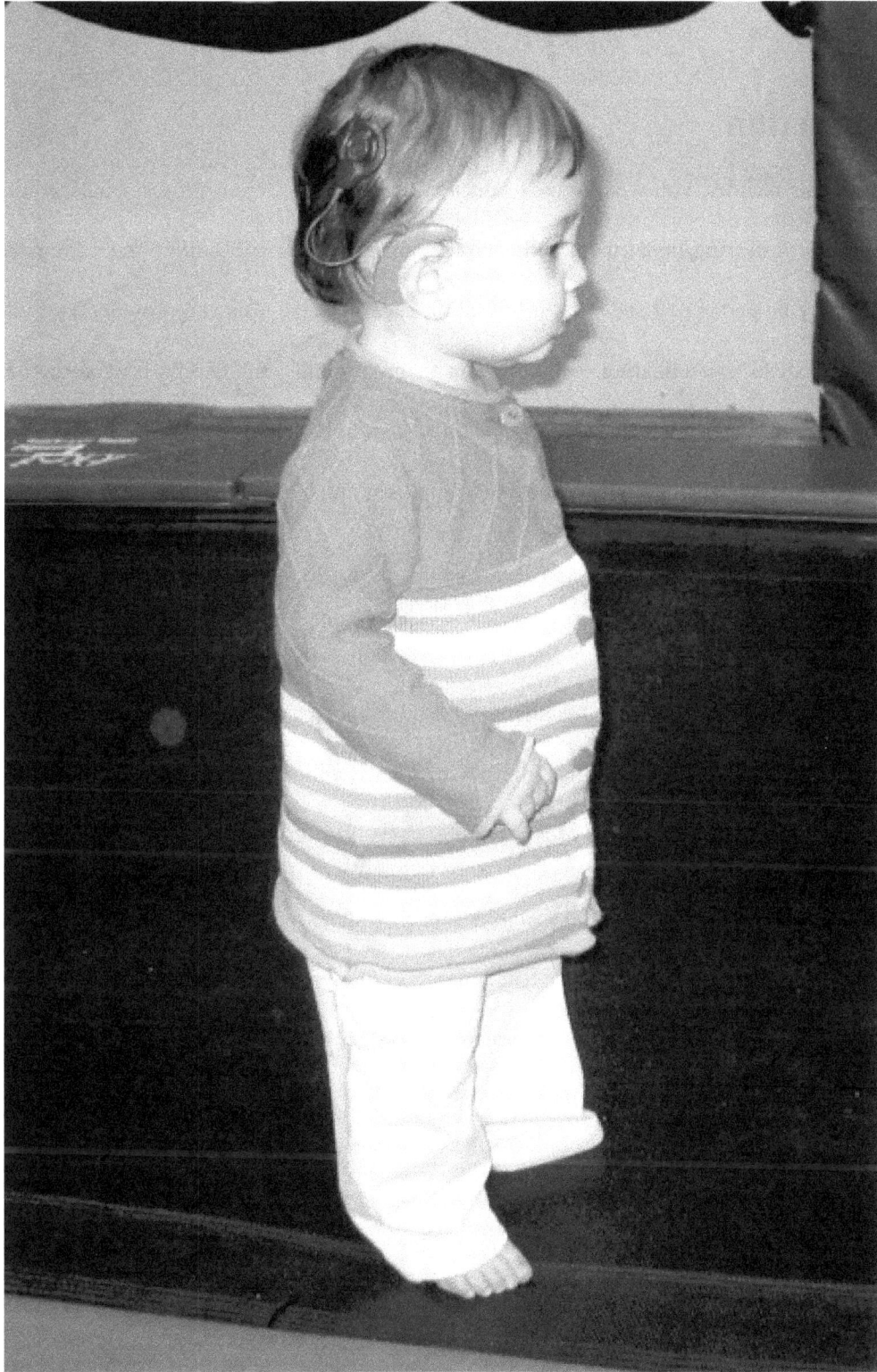

Introduction

In this chapter, you will become educated about the different professionals involved in the diagnosis of hearing impairment and each of their roles. We will outline the various hearing tests that may be performed and what information each of those tests can provide. You will also learn how to read an audiogram, enabling you to understand your child's hearing test results. With knowledge comes empowerment to take on a seemingly daunting task. We are here to equip you with the knowledge and tools necessary to help your child.

Your Support Team

Your very first decisions in the process of addressing your child's hearing impairment begin with the care group you put together—your draft choices to build the team of professionals you direct. You will begin by finding the professionals who can help you determine the exact level of hearing impairment and its cause.

This process requires several specialists, each with a separate set of technical abilities and with knowledge you will need. Each team member should be providing you not only with a service, but also with knowledge, judgment, and advice. Remembering this will help you understand the purpose and goals of each interaction with the treatment team members as you go forward.

For example, a physician specializing in the ear can advise you in areas such as which treatment strategies are most likely to produce the best language development for your child. This same professional can also provide services as simple as cleaning wax from the ear, or as complex as placing a cochlear implant, should it be necessary.

There is some overlap in knowledge that these professionals can share; however, in most urban settings you can find each of these specialists, though not always under a single roof. In some cases, you may need to go out of town for services. Occasionally, families will choose to relocate to an area more fitting to their children's needs.

Your best and fastest source of information may be parents of children with hearing impairments living in your area. You can find these families online through Internet support groups. If you can, contact several support groups, either in person or electronically. You will find that experiences, goals, and the situations of different children affect the advice and opinions of different families. Some areas have face-to-face support groups for hearing-impaired individuals and their families. The vast majority of parents of children with hearing impairments are delighted to share their advice and experience—and you may be too, when another family contacts you in the future.

Pediatric Audiologist

A pediatric audiologist specializes in hearing testing and rehabilitation of hearing in infants and children. In addition to hearing testing, pediatric audiologists are trained to restore hearing using electronic means such as hearing aids and other similar technology. These professionals are an excellent source of information regarding appropriate nonmedical therapy, such as speech and language therapy and/or auditory training. The pediatric audiologist can also counsel you on the impact of hearing loss in educational settings and how to minimize that impact, as well as inform you of many other services that will be needed.

The **knowledge/judgment** a pediatric audiologist should be able to contribute includes:

- Whether treatment is needed and when it should begin
- What nonmedical treatments are appropriate

- Which hearing device (a hearing aid, assistive listening device, or cochlear implant) is best for your child

- What educational, therapy, and treatment options are available locally

   Services provided by a pediatric audiologist include:

- Hearing testing and occasionally balance testing, as this is also a function of the inner ear and can be an issue in some types of hearing impairment

- Selection, maintenance, and programming of hearing aids

- In conjunction with an ear physician: selection, maintenance, and programming of cochlear implants (a special ability found in a cochlear implant audiologist)

In some cases, you may see one audiologist to diagnose your child's hearing impairment (diagnostic audiology), while a separate individual selects and programs the hearing device (treating audiology). A further subspecialty of audiology is educational audiology, which involves making recommendations about a child's educational setting with respect to special equipment needed, classroom acoustics, assessment testing, and remediation.

Your relationship with your pediatric audiologist will be long lasting, with multiple visits at regular intervals. Because you will need to see this individual frequently, you may need to factor convenience and availability into your selection decision. Make very sure this provider is the best you can find. Your child's result will depend heavily on the audiologist's services and advice.

Educators/Therapists

The role of the educator/therapist is to evaluate your child's communication and cognitive development level, and also to intervene when needed to assist in producing optimal results. Several titles exist for educators and therapists who play different roles in the treatment of hearing impairment. Educators and therapists can include:

- Speech/language pathologists

- Auditory oral therapists

- Auditory verbal therapists

- Deaf educators

- Developmental psychologists

- Occupational therapists

- Counselors

The **knowledge/judgment** that educators and therapists should be able to contribute includes the ability to identify and communicate where your child is in his or her developmental progress in terms of speech and language, cognitive development, school performance, motor development, and/or any other aspect of normal pediatric development that they specialize in; and the ability to recommend interventions with the goal of advancing your child's development toward his or her highest potential. It is important not to sabotage a hearing-impaired child by setting low expectations based on the hearing impairment alone.

Services provided by educators and therapists include the teaching and supervision of training exercises used to develop any area of human performance. For example, speech and language therapists will work with your child to aid in the development of vocabulary, reading skills, comprehension, pronunciation and articulation, and other communication skills. Occupational therapists will work on motor development, such as coordination, balance, and fine motor skills. Think of these individuals as very specialized teachers for your hearing-impaired child.

Clearly, you will not be able to find all needed educator/therapist skills in one person.

You may, however, be able find them in a single location that employs multiple individuals, such as a children's hospital. Commonly, a team of people in different locations may be drafted over time to help you and your child achieve your goals.

Your team will change over time as different needs are addressed at different developmental stages. For example, in the early years, the primary focus may be development of speech production skills, while reading and motor development become more central during the early school years. Remember, you are the constant for your child. You are the coach, and you remain in charge of this team.

There is no formula to determine how much time your child needs from each type of therapist. Some children need no intervention in certain areas. Others, even with the same hearing loss and diagnosis, need quite a bit. There are as many solutions as there are children with hearing impairment.

Your team of hearing health care professionals will give you their input, and you need to decide what is needed and what will be best for your child. For this reason, the process of defining and applying the appropriate education and therapy program for a hearing-impaired child needs to be watched closely and almost continuously over a long period of time. The trick is to stay on top of the changing needs of your child and to address each area before a big problem emerges.

Some services may be needed for a long period of time. In general, however, the most intense developmental training for children with hearing impairments is in the preschool age group, because of the crucial period of language development that occurs during this time. It is a much better strategy to provide the needed input during the key brain development window for certain skills rather than trying to play catch-up later.

Some educational/therapy services may be available and paid for through governmental organizations or schools, while others may be covered through your health insurance. However, some services will likely require significant financial contributions from the family.

Ear Physician

Physicians who specialize in the medical treatment and surgical evaluation of ear disorders are known as ear, nose, and throat (ENT) specialists, or otolaryngologists. A select group of ENT specialists receive further training in the areas of hearing and balance disorders during an additional two-year fellowship. These professionals are called otologists and focus solely on the ear.

Several hundred disorders and syndromes include hearing impairment as one factor; the ear physician's knowledge of these syndromes is critical to determine whether other issues besides hearing impairment are or will be present in your child.

The **knowledge/judgment** that an ear physician should be able to contribute includes:

- What treatment is needed, if any, and when it should begin

- Where certain diagnostic services and treatment are available

- What educational, therapy, and treatment options are available locally

- What other medical professionals are needed in the evaluation or treatment of your child, to whom the ear physician can provide referrals

- When to use a cochlear implant and which device to choose if it is needed

Services provided by an ear physician include:

- Diagnosing the hearing impairment, its cause, and any related syndromes

- Evaluating and treating the balance system if necessary

- Stabilizing or improving hearing in some patients through medical or surgical intervention

- Keeping the ear functioning as well as possible—for example, by cleaning wax, treating recurrent infections, or removing middle ear fluid

- Performing surgical placement of a cochlear implant or implantable hearing aid if needed

- Follow-up monitoring of hearing impairment over time in order to identify medical conditions that may show up when your child is older

- Applying new diagnostic and treatment options for hearing impairment as they emerge over time

If possible, it is best to find an ear physician and pediatric audiologist who are accustomed to working together, preferably located in the same facility. In many situations, both professionals are needed on the same day. For example, a typical clinic visit may include wax removal followed by a hearing test with a diagnostic audiologist, followed by a device adjustment by the same or a different treating audiologist, followed by a medical follow-up to discuss surgery or medicinal options. Travelling between different sites for this series of services can be very inconvenient, time-consuming, and costly; and most important, it can result in critical delays in treatment if the pediatric audiologist, ear physician, and educational audiologist do not agree on a treatment plan.

Hearing impairment evaluation and treatment is a rapidly changing field, with new knowledge that affects clinical practice almost constantly. When choosing an ear physician, look for a special interest and focus on hearing impairment in children, up-to-date knowledge in the field, clinical experience, availability, and a convenient location. Expect to visit this professional less frequently than your pediatric audiologist, most likely somewhere between two and six times per year. In most cases, your ear physician will be needed more in the early phases of diagnosis and treatment. Later on, some appointments will involve only the pediatric audiologist.

Surgical ability and patient outcomes may become important as time goes by if your child needs surgery. You may find that your regular ear physician has the requisite skills, or you may decide to go to a specialized center for certain surgical services.

Geneticist/Genetic Counselor

A geneticist is trained in the evaluation and diagnosis of genetically transmitted diseases. Hearing impairment is caused by a genetic abnormality in a high percentage of patients.

The **knowledge/judgment** that a geneticist should be able to contribute includes:

- Understanding the genetic causes responsible for hearing impairment, including other symptoms of the genetic abnormality if one exists

- Identifying other, non-hearing-related symptoms of certain genetically caused disorders

Services provided by a geneticist include:

- Testing for genetic causes responsible for hearing impairment

- Identifying other, non-hearing-related symptoms of certain genetic abnormalities

- Assessing the risk that future children of yours will have the same genetic abnormality if one exists

- Assessing the risk that your child's children will have the same genetic abnormality if one exists

What to Look For

Your ear physician will guide you to geneticists in your area. If you are from a small area, you may need to travel to a large center if counseling is needed. In most situations, your ear physician can order needed tests to determine if a genetic cause of hearing impairment exists. If a genetic cause is found, then it is time to consider genetic counseling. Many pediatricians are also very skilled in genetic counseling.

This is an area where knowledge is currently exploding, and it will continue to do so over the next several decades. Currently, only diagnosis is available for a growing number of genetic causes of hearing impairment. In the future, it is likely that treatment will become available for some conditions as well.

Pediatrician

A pediatrician is a physician specializing in the general health needs of children.

The **knowledge/judgment** that a pediatrician should be able to contribute includes an understanding of the normal and abnormal functional and developmental status of children.

Services provided by a pediatrician include treatment of ear infections and other illnesses that may affect the function of the ears during childhood, and evaluation of non-hearing systems for evidence of abnormality. This needs to happen over time, as some organ system abnormalities associated with hearing impairment will not show up for many months or years.

What to Look For

Every child needs a pediatrician for health maintenance, immunizations, treatment of the usual childhood illnesses, etc. Coordination between the pediatrician and the ear physician will be necessary to keep the ears functioning at the best of their ability. For example, a simple ear infection produces a temporary hearing impairment due to fluid in the middle ear. If your child already has a hearing impairment and additional hearing impairment is added from a middle ear infection, hearing function may be severely impacted. As a result, your child will need more aggressive treatment of ear infections. Most ear physicians work with a very wide range of pediatricians in their geographic areas.

Try not to be overwhelmed by the list of professionals covered here. You do not need everyone in place immediately, and some of those discussed here may be needed only for a very short time—or perhaps not at all.

The two most important players that all families with a child with a suspected hearing impairment need as soon as possible are a *pediatric audiologist* and an *ear physician*. These two professionals will allow you to answer the following questions:

1. Is there a hearing impairment, and if so, what is the type and level of loss?
2. What caused the hearing impairment, and what can be done to reverse it or prevent it from getting worse?
3. What treatment options are available, and what are the benefits and downsides of each option?

Your pediatric audiologist and your ear physician will guide you in determining the next series of questions needed to put together the team for your child.

Hearing Tests

Once a hearing impairment is suspected, several questions need to be answered as soon as possible. These include whether hearing impairment is present and the type and severity of the hearing impairment. The earlier these questions are answered, the earlier a child can begin treatment, often resulting in better outcomes in speech and language development. Remember the critical period in childhood language development? If you follow out-of-date advice to wait until your child is older to get more accurate test results, the delay in diagnosing and treating your child's hearing impairment may result in lifelong language delays. Hearing can be tested at any age *if the testing facility you select has the right objective testing equipment and personnel.* If the testing facility you select tells you that they are unable to test your child's hearing, find another facility.

Your pediatric audiologist will use one or more of the following tests to determine whether your child has a hearing impairment. In most cases, more than one test may be necessary to be 100 percent certain of the presence, type, and severity of hearing impairment. This is particularly true with tests designed to be screening evaluations. In addition, tests may be repeated several times, either to confirm the findings of the first test or, in the case of progressive hearing impairments, which can get worse over time, to chart the course of the progression.

Not all children who receive referrals after infant hearing screening are found to have hearing impairments. Each screening program has a small percentage of children referred for further testing who are subsequently found to have normal hearing.

Hearing testing in very young children requires experienced, highly trained, and talented pediatric audiologists and otologists, as well as very expensive and delicate equipment. Many hearing centers lack the facilities, personnel, or equipment to conduct all the types of objective tests listed here. Because the results of these tests are crucial for diagnosing and treating hearing impairment, it is essential to travel, if necessary, to a facility where this type of testing is performed on a routine basis.

Hearing testing falls into one of two categories: subjective testing and objective testing. Subjective testing relies on the child to respond to a sound. The test subject must show some type of behavior to the examining pediatric audiologist, which indicates that the sound was heard. In older children who are able to follow simple instructions, subjective tests can be performed through a traditional "raise your hand when you hear the beep" test. In younger children and individuals who cannot yet communicate, pediatric audiologists use behavior to determine which sounds the child is responding to. Subjective testing can be used with older children and adults and requires a participating, alert test subject.

Objective testing does not rely on any information or expressive reaction by the subject being tested. The pediatric audiologist uses measurements of electrical responses generated by the patient's hearing system and/or brain to determine if sound is being received and processed. As you may guess, very young infants need objective testing. Generally speaking, children must be very soundly asleep for optimal objective testing results. In infants, this testing can sometimes be coordinated around naptime or in combination with over-the-counter medication known to cause drowsiness, such as Benadryl. In some cases, sedation or even general anesthesia may be required to complete objective testing.

Subjective Testing

There are several types of subjective testing for hearing impairment. The audiologist will consider the following factors to determine which type of test is most suitable for any given patient:

1. The age of the patient
2. The expressive and receptive communication abilities of the patient
3. Any other medical conditions the patient may have that might interfere with the hearing test examination

Conventional Audiometry

The most commonly used subjective hearing test is the conventional audiogram. A complete audiogram includes testing of the following parameters:

- Bone conduction, which indicates how well the child hears when sound is directly conducted through the skull

- Air conduction, which indicates how well the child hears when sound is conducted through the ear

- Immittance testing, which tests the function of the eardrum and middle ear structures

- Speech discrimination testing

Conventional audiometry testing begins with a measure of air conduction thresholds. Air conduction measures the sound heard through the ear canal. A sound-emitting probe is placed in the ear canal, or headphones are placed over the ears. By individual frequency, the pediatric audiologist identifies the softest sound the test subject is able to hear at each frequency. If the test subject hears the sound, he or she communicates this to the pediatric audiologist, usually by pressing an indicator button or raising a hand. Each ear is tested on its own.

Next, bone conduction thresholds are measured using a vibrating device, which is placed firmly against the skin of the forehead or the bone behind the ear, called the mastoid. Sounds are sent as vibrations from this device and are carried through the bone of the skull directly to the inner ear. Inner ear nerve fibers, known as hair cells, receive the sounds and turn them into electrical impulses before transmitting the signal to the brain. Bone conduction measures the ability of the hearing nerve to receive sound. A reduced or absent ability of the hearing nerve to receive sound indicates the presence of a sensorineural hearing impairment.

When the sound-collecting system of the ear (the outer ear, ear canal, eardrum, and middle ear bones) is working properly, bone conduction and air conduction testing results will be identical. When air conduction testing results show that sound must be louder to be heard as compared to bone conduction, it is clear that the sound-collecting system of the ear is not working perfectly. This condition is known as a conductive hearing impairment. Air conduction hearing results can never be better than bone conduction hearing results.

In summary, hearing impairment can be **sensorineural** (due to a hearing nerve problem), **conductive** (due to dysfunction of the sound-collecting system of the middle and outer ear), or **mixed,** with both sensorineural and conductive components.

Obviously, this type of test requires participation and cooperation from the test subject. As a generalization, the earliest conventional audiometry can be attempted is in the five- to six-year age range.

Tympanogram

Immittance testing uses a pressure-producing probe placed in the ear canal. Immittance testing results are recorded in a graph called a tympanogram. The test is quick and painless. It can be done in even the youngest infants, and the patient does not have to be asleep. In some cases, a rare condition called canal stenosis will prevent this test from being performed. The equipment used to conduct immittance testing consists of three parts: a tiny loudspeaker to produce sound waves, a microphone to pick up the response, and an air pump.

By varying the pressure of the ear canal in both positive and negative directions while measuring sound bounced off the tympanic membrane (or eardrum), the health of the middle ear space can be determined. Normal middle ear space is only filled with air, which allows the eardrum to vibrate correctly. Fluid or any other material in the middle ear space will restrict those vibrations. If fluid is present in the middle ear, this will result in a conductive hearing impairment, which will generate an abnormal tympanogram. If a pressure equalization (PE) tube is present, the tympanogram can show whether the tubes are open. In addition, the function of two small muscles attached to the middle ear bones can be tested with the immittance probe. This test will provide information about the cause of certain types of conductive hearing impairments.

Conditioned Play Audiometry

Conditioned play audiometry (CPA) uses the same basic testing parameters as described above for conventional audiometry; however, this type of testing is intended for children from two and a half to four years of age. CPA testing involves conditioning a child to perform a task when he or she hears a sound. For example, the pediatric audiologist may condition the child to throw a ball in a bucket or place a peg on a board when he or she hears a sound. This form of testing is more interesting for a young child than a conventional hand-raising test, and can produce more accurate, reliable results when done correctly.

Visual Reinforcement Audiometry

Visual reinforcement audiometry (VRA) utilizes the same basic testing parameters as described above for CPA. However, an essential component of VRA testing involves conditioning a child to look toward the sound source when a sound occurs. When the child looks toward the sound, an interesting and pleasing toy is activated as a reward. The toy generally involves motion and lights. Once the initial training has been accomplished, the pediatric audiologist can tell when the child hears a sound because the child will turn toward the sound or toy in anticipation of its activation.

VRA requires a skilled pediatric audiologist who is able to vary presentation times enough to differentiate between a true response and a false positive. Many times, the child will constantly look back and forth between speakers in the hope of catching the toy. This looking may happen to coincide with the pediatric audiologist's presentation of sound, and could be recorded as a true response when in fact the child did not hear the sound. For this reason, children younger than three years of age will often be scheduled with two audiologists or an audiologist and a test assistant. The test assistant or second audiologist will sit in front of the child in order to keep his or her attention forward, and may also help the pediatric audiologist to identify a true response.

VRA testing can generally be performed in children from six months to three years of age.

Behavioral Observation Audiometry

Behavioral observation audiometry (BOA) utilizes the same parameters as described above for conventional audiometry. However, rather than the patient (who is usually an infant) responding to the examiner with words or with hand motions, the pediatric audiologist is looking for some type of behavioral reaction indicating that the child has heard the sound. This response may be as subtle as eye widening, a pause in sucking, or a head turn. BOA testing can generally be performed with children from six months to three years of age. A combination of BOA and VRA can be used if the patient is not completely reliable in one form only. A test assistant is typically used with this form of testing, as well.

CPA, VRA, and BOA testing can be inaccurate, and results are highly dependent on the mood, sleepiness, fussiness, etc., of the child, as well as the experience of the examiner and the testing assistant.

Speech Discrimination Testing

Speech discrimination ability is assessed by presenting age-appropriate word, phrase, or sentence lists to the test subject. The test subject then repeats the spoken utterance that he or she believes was heard, and its accuracy is graded. Accuracy is scored based on both words and phonemes, the smallest unit of a word. For example, if the audiologist said "rake" but the patient repeated "rate," she would be scored 0 for words (because the word she repeated was incorrect) and 2 out of 3 for phonemes— because she got the "r" and "a" phonemes correct, but repeated the ending of the word incorrectly. Since infants and young children have little or no expressive or receptive language development, this test is usually of more value in children over six years of age and adults.

Objective Testing

Objective hearing testing involves tests that require no conscious feedback or communication skills from the individual being tested. They are perfect, therefore, for children who are too young to communicate, or for individuals who have other medical issues, such as autism, that may make subjective testing impossible to perform reliably.

Automated Auditory Brainstem Response (Infant Hearing Screening Testing)

Our brain reacts to sound even when we are asleep. Infant hearing screening capitalizes on this fact by making clicking noises at various decibel (loudness) levels and in various frequencies, then measuring the infant's responses to those sounds.

Infant hearing screening programs use extremely limited testing. These tests, which are frequently conducted in the newborn nursery setting, are designed only to determine whether the patient is responding to sound presented in what is considered a normal hearing range.

Infant hearing screening program testing utilizes recording electrodes that are placed on the skin and are designed to record very small electrical currents. A clicking sound is directed into the ear canal via a small insert. This clicking sound is meant to stimulate the hearing nerve pathway at a low intensity, like that of a soft voice. When the infant hears this sound, even while asleep, the hearing pathway fires off very small electrical charges, which are sensed by the surface electrodes (see Figure 2-1).

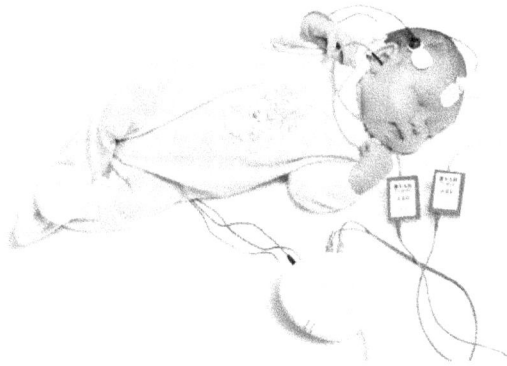

Figure 2-1
Copyright © MAICO Diagnostic

Recording equipment attached to the surface electrodes records the response, which presents as a waveform. A normal human auditory pathway produces very standardized waveforms. An automated computerized system compares the waveforms produced to known normal waveforms.

Infants do not "fail" infant hearing screenings. They either pass, meaning the waveform that is generated is considered to be a normal waveform response to the sound being presented (indicating normal hearing), or they are referred for more thorough testing procedures. Unfortunately, infant hearing screening is associated with a high number of false positive results. False positives occur when it is thought that the child might be hearing-impaired but it later turns out that he or she has normal hearing. The most frequent cause of false positives is fluid behind the middle ear, causing a temporary conductive hearing impairment. The second most common cause of false positives is the infant not being completely asleep when the test starts, or waking up in the middle of the test. It is absolutely essential that the infant be asleep for the infant hearing screening results to be valid.

Auditory Brainstem Response (ABR)

An ABR is the most commonly used investigation to determine if a hearing impairment is present. This is frequently the next examination performed after a child receives a "referral" result from the infant hearing screening test. ABR testing produces results by generating several hundred broadband sound clicks and recording the responses, then producing a measurable waveform from those results. The ABR equipment can test hearing with sound levels up to 90 decibels. However, ABRs cannot provide information about each specific frequency represented on the audiogram.

ABR examinations also use surface electrodes and sensitive recording equipment to record an electrical waveform produced in the hearing pathway. Once sound enters the inner ear, nerve stimulation begins in the cochlea and proceeds up the hearing pathway through several following nerve centers to the conscious level, where we become aware of the sound. The entire process takes only a fraction of a second.

If the test is performed with special techniques using narrow-band sound clicks, the pediatric audiologist can focus the investigation on specific hearing frequencies—either high or low. The size, timing, and onset of the waveform can give information about how several different areas of the auditory pathway are functioning. A coordinated firing of nerve cells has to occur in order to produce clear and understandable speech to the brain. Poor coordination of nerve signals is easily identifiable on an ABR. An ABR can help to gain information about mild, moderate, and some severe hearing impairment. If the patient's hearing impairment is greater than 90 decibels, no waveform will be generated at all.

Since the test measures tiny electrical impulses, and since electrical impulses are also generated with muscle movement, the test subject must be very still during the test. For all practical purposes, this can only be accomplished during sleep or sedation. In most cases, very young children can have the test performed during a nap. Children who may have trouble staying still will need sedation, or occasionally general anesthesia, for test accuracy. Test duration is generally one to two hours, depending on how well the child sleeps, and requires the pediatric audiologist to identify the correct waveforms.

Because colds, ear infections, and allergies can all cause congestion, resulting in temporary conductive hearing impairment, an ABR performed when one of these conditions exists may generate inaccurate results.

Here is a practical but simplified explanation of how an ABR test is executed. The test frequently begins by generating sound at 60 decibels. If the waveform is flat, then the child cannot hear sound at 60 decibels, and thus his or her hearing threshold must be higher than 60 decibels. The pediatric audiologist then increases the loudness of the sound at 5-decibel increments until either the 90-decibel maximum level is reached, or a waveform is produced.

If a normal waveform exists at 60 decibels, then the child can hear sound at 60 decibels, and thus his or her hearing threshold must be lower than 60 decibels. The pediatric audiologist then decreases the loudness of the sound level in 5-decibel steps. If a hearing impairment is present, the ABR waveform will decrease in size until it completely disappears at the level of the child's hearing impairment. If there is still a normal waveform at 20 decibels, that is considered hearing within normal limits. An ABR from a child with normal hearing is shown below (Figure 2-2).

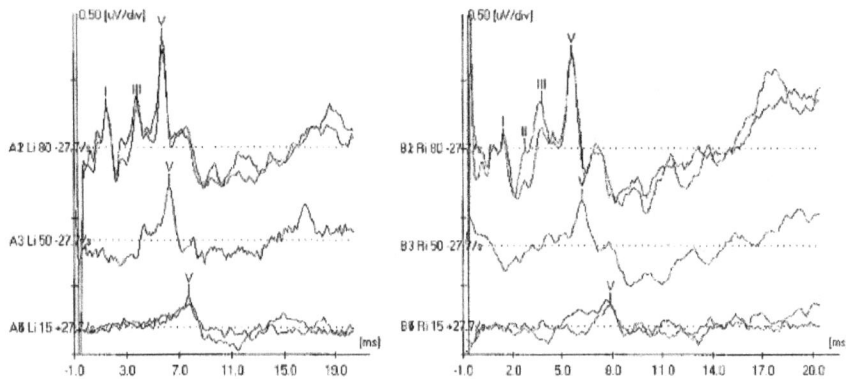

Figure 2-2 Example of a normal ABR

Auditory Steady-State Response

An auditory steady-state response (ASSR) examination is somewhat similar to an ABR examination, in that both hearing tests use sound-producing probes and surface recording electrodes. ASSR is a newer technology that has been commercially available in the United States since it received FDA approval in July of 2001. Instead of presenting sound using broad- or narrow-band sound clicks, an ASSR uses sound at each frequency, which is varied in intensity and warbled to slightly lower and higher frequencies simultaneously. Sophisticated computer analysis of the waveforms produced records the data in an audiogram format, which can be seen in Figure 2-3.

The information from an ASSR examination provides nearly all of the same information generated by an ABR examination, plus several types of additional information. An ASSR examination can present a broader range of sound, with a maximum of 120 decibels, as opposed to the 90-decibel limit of the ABR examination. Therefore, the ASSR examination is the only test that reliably generates accurate results for patients whose hearing impairment is suspected to be in the "profound" range. In addition, the ASSR can provide more detailed information about the specific frequencies of the hearing impairment. This is extremely important, because hearing impairment curves are generally not flat and often have some type of slope, either downward, upward, or a combination of the two. Having more specific information about the level of hearing impairment associated with each frequency is indispensable in determining which type of treatment to select, and for programming certain devices used for treatment.

Like the ABR, the ASSR test requires the subject to be very still. ASSR testing can be performed faster than ABR testing, usually requiring one hour to complete. Not all centers currently have this technology available with adequately trained pediatric audiologists.

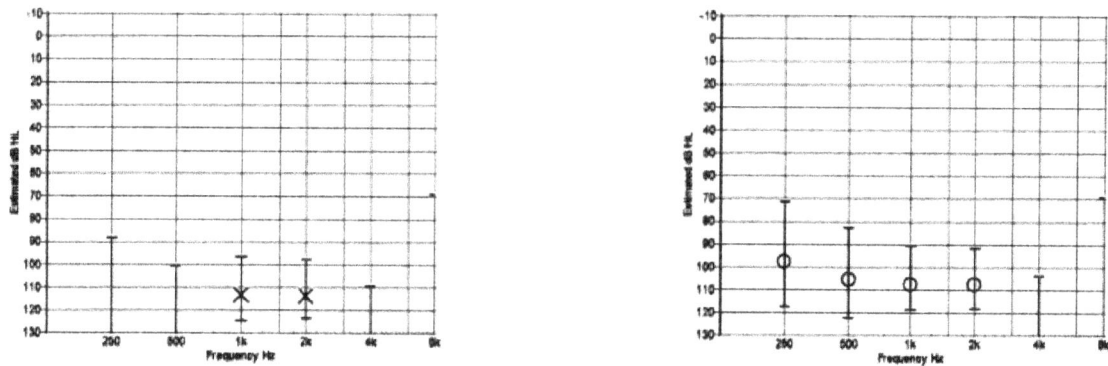

Figure 2-3 Example of ASSR results

Otoacoustic Emissions

Nerve receptor cells (called hair cells) in the cochlea take the vibrational sound energy transmitted to the inner ear by the eardrum and middle ear bones and turn it into electrical impulses. The hair cells transmit the electrical energy to the auditory pathway, where it is carried to the brain for processing. As the hair cells receive and transform the vibrational energy, they "twitch." The tiny hair cell twitches produce a miniscule sound, which is transmitted in reverse from the inner ear, through the middle ear bones and back out to the eardrum, where it is released into the ear canal. The sound produced by the tiny hair cell twitches is far too small to hear with our own ears. However, very delicate instruments can not only detect, but also measure this sound.

Think of an old submarine movie where the sonar man sends out a "ping" and waits for the sound to return. In a very basic way, that's what the otoacoustic emissions (OAE) test does. When the returning ping (or otoacoustic emission) is detected, it means that the twitching hair cells are present and active. As most sensorineural hearing impairment involves some disorder of hair cell function, this is extremely useful information. In a practical sense, if an otoacoustic emission is heard, we know the patient has hearing in the 0- to 25-decibel range, generally considered within normal limits.

OAE testing is an essential component of diagnosing a type of hearing impairment known as auditory neuropathy, which is the source of approximately 3 percent of all infant hearing impairment in the United States.

The OAE test is quick and painless, and it gives information at each frequency band. It requires a still, quiet patient. However, several sources of error can cause inaccurate OAE test results. For example, fluid in the middle ear will dampen the sound generated by the tiny otoacoustic emission, resulting in an absent response. The audiologist may misinterpret the results as indicating an inner ear hearing impairment. Therefore, it is very important for your child to be checked for middle ear fluid by a qualified physician prior to proceeding with this examination.

Figure 2-4 is an example of OAE test results for the left ear.

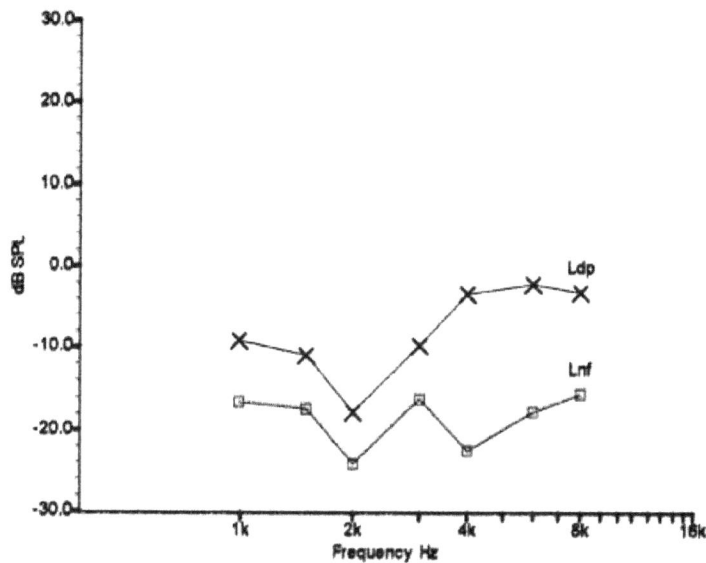

Figure 2-4 Example of DPOAE results for the left ear

Types of Hearing Impairment

It is important to understand what type of hearing impairment is present in order to understand which treatment options and devices are most appropriate and what outcome is most likely.

There are two major types of hearing impairment: sensorineural and conductive. Sensorineural hearing impairment is the most common type. It indicates a condition in which the sound is reaching the cochlea, but for whatever reason, the sound is not reaching the brain to be processed. Conductive hearing impairment exists when the sound is being blocked before it can reach the cochlea, either due to a temporary blockage such as wax or fluid, or a permanent blockage due to some congenital deformity, cyst, or issue with the middle ear bones or the eardrum.

It is important to know whether the hearing impairment is conductive or sensorineural for several reasons:

1. Conductive hearing impairment has a maximum of 55 decibels, while sensorineural hearing impairment has no maximum.

2. Conductive loss, depending on the source, can be temporary.

3. Conductive loss, depending on the source, can occasionally be surgically corrected without the use of any hearing devices or cochlear implants.

4. Different hearing aids are better suited for conductive losses than for sensorineural losses.

When both conductive and sensorineural hearing impairment exists, this is referred to as a "mixed" type of hearing impairment.

A fourth, rarer form of hearing impairment is **central hearing impairment, sometimes referred to as auditory neuropathy, which** results from impaired nerves or nuclei of the central nervous system, either in the pathways to the brain or in the brain itself.

Finally, another extremely rare form of hearing impairment is completely absent eighth cranial (auditory) nerves. Individuals with absent auditory nerves cannot benefit from cochlear implants. A related surgical procedure, known as an auditory brainstem implant, can provide these individuals with some sound awareness; however, the ability to recognize speech is unlikely.

In addition to the previously noted types of hearing impairment, hearing impairment can either be stable or progressive. A progressive hearing impairment is one that gets worse over time. Some disorders known to cause hearing impairment, such as enlarged vestibular aqueducts, cytomegalovirus, and Usher's syndrome, are known to be progressive in nature.

Levels of Hearing Impairment

The level of hearing impairment is defined based on the lowest level of sound that the individual is able to hear. This is measured in units known as decibels, frequently abbreviated as dB. While there is some variation in the labeling associated with different levels of hearing impairment, the most typical categorization is as follows:

Normal hearing: For adults: between 0 and 25 dB

                                           For children: between 0 and 20 dB

Mild hearing impairment: For adults: between 26 and 40 dB

                                           For children: between 21 and 40 dB

Moderate hearing impairment: Between 41 and 55 dB

Moderately severe hearing impairment: Between 56 and 70 dB

Severe hearing impairment: Between 71 and 90 dB

Profound hearing impairment: 91 dB or greater

How to Read Hearing Test Results

Now look at Figure 2-5. This is an audiogram, and you need to understand how to interpret it. Almost all hearing test results, both subjective and objective, are displayed in an audiogram format. The vertical lines (A) are the individual frequencies, which are labeled across the top of the audiogram. You see that frequencies tested range from 250 Hz to 8,000 Hz. The majority of speech falls in the 500- to 4,000-Hz range. The horizontal lines (B) are the volume levels. They are labeled along the left side of the graph from 0 to 120 decibels. Zero decibels does not mean there is no sound, but is defined as the lowest level at which those with perfect hearing can perceive the tone tested. One-hundred twenty decibels is a very loud sound, in the range of gunfire or jet engine noise. Normal hearing is defined as the ability to hear 0 to 20 decibels and above in children and 0 to 25 decibels and above in adults.

Bone conduction and air conduction are graphed with different symbols, as you see in the audiogram key (C). Tympanograms are reported in a separate area (D). Speech discrimination testing is shown in the area between right and left ear bone and air conduction testing results (E). Lastly, middle ear muscle function, called acoustic reflex testing, is shown in a separate area (F).

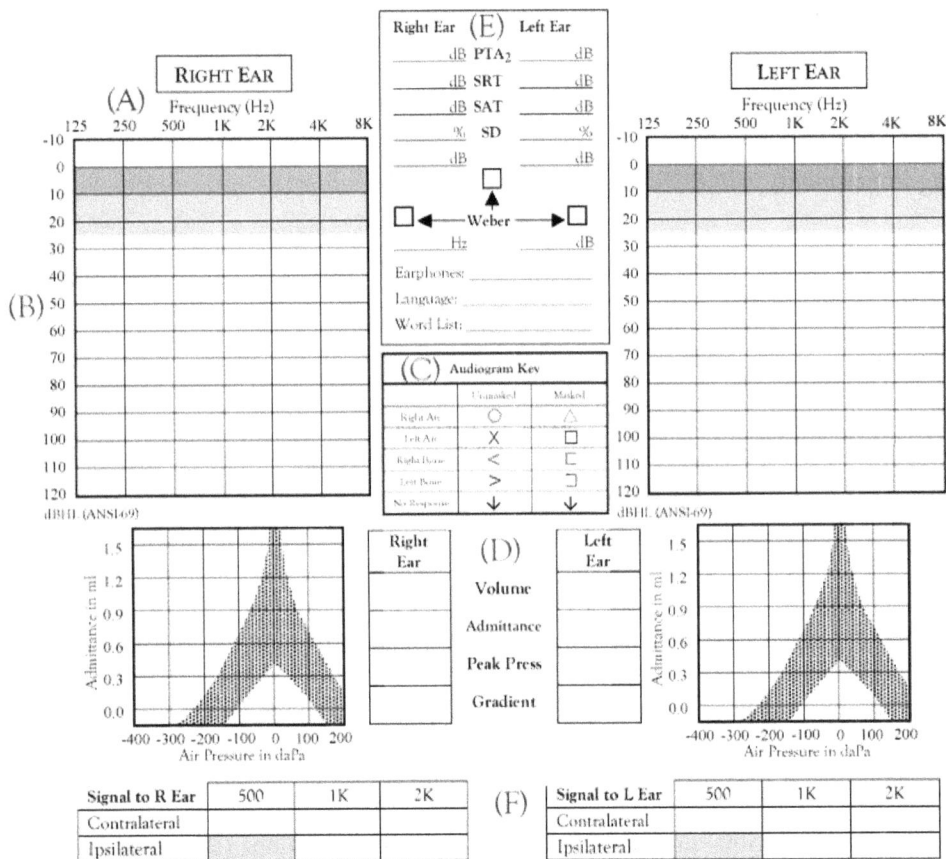

Figure 2-5 Audiogram

Figures 2-6 through 2-9 give you some examples of audiograms showing normal hearing and various types of hearing impairments.

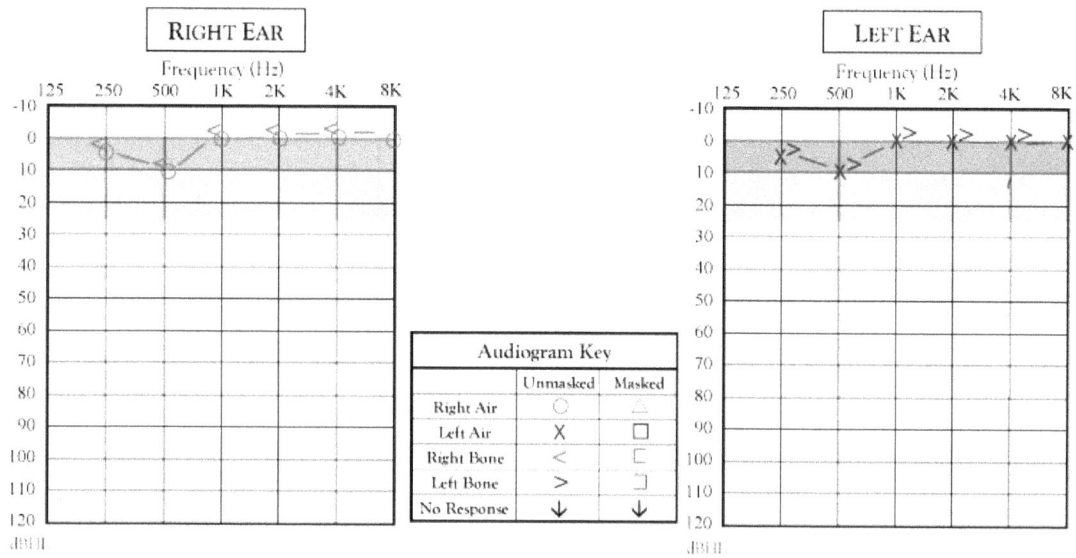

Figure 2-6 Example of normal audiogram

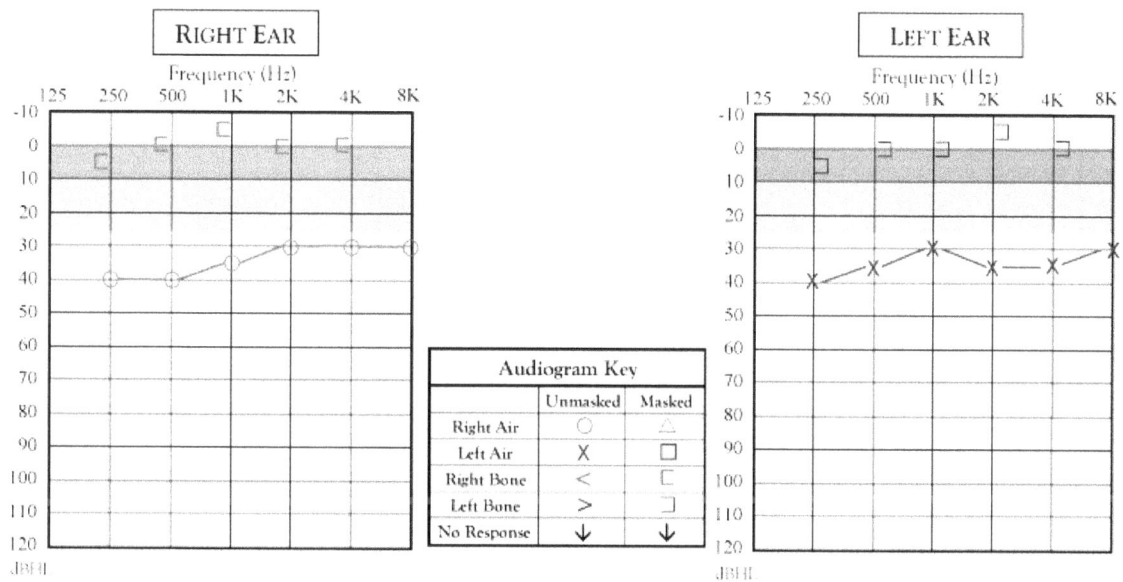

Figure 2-7 Example of bilateral conductive hearing impairment

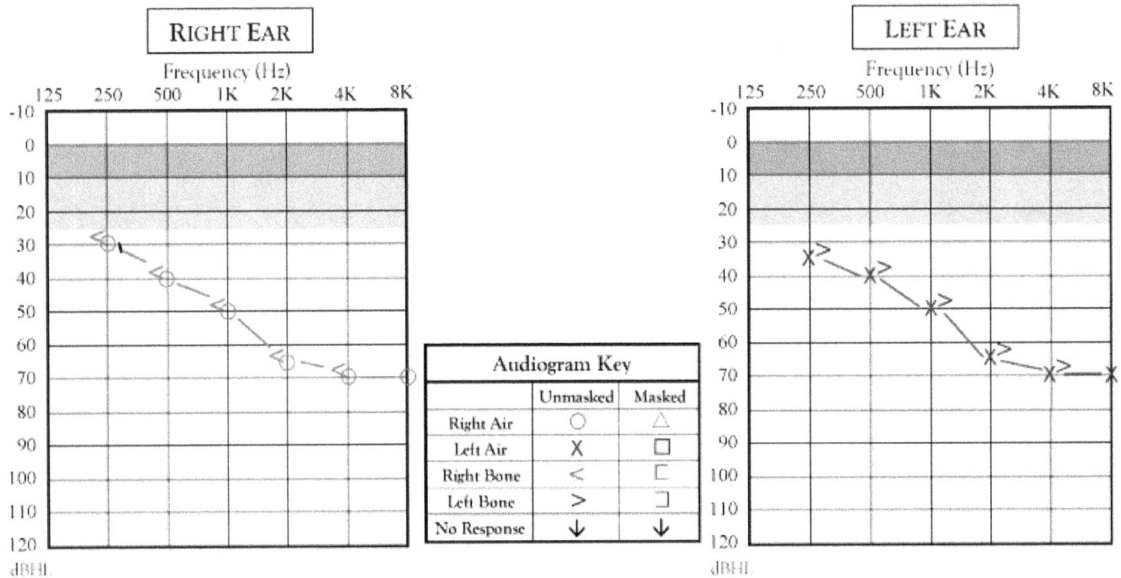

Figure 2-8 Example of bilateral sensorineural hearing impairment

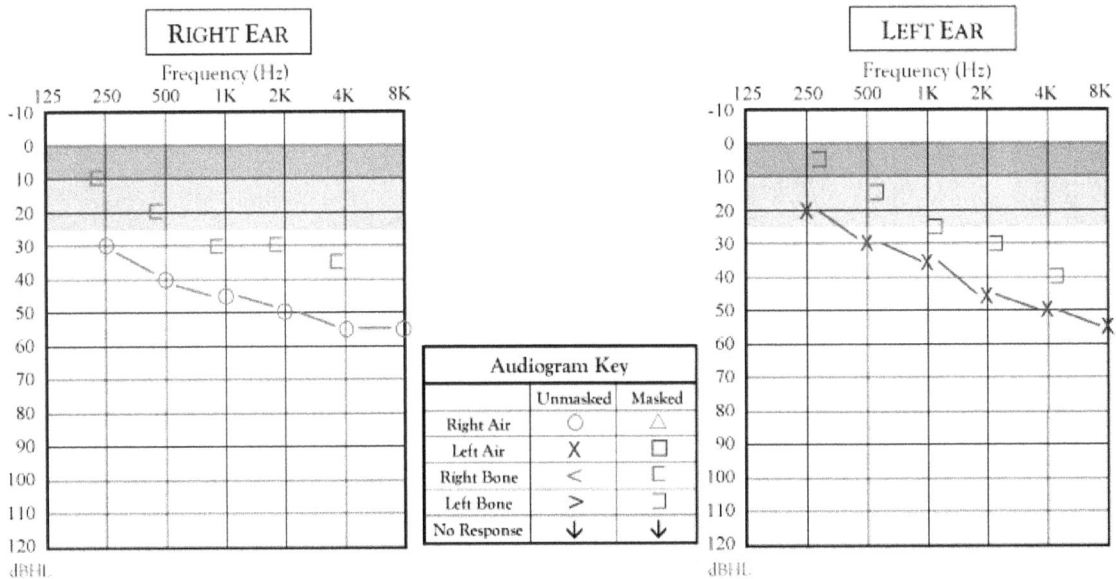

Figure 2-9 Example of bilateral mixed hearing impairment

There is one last descriptive categorization of hearing impairment that you need to understand. The severity of hearing impairment can be described as mild, moderate, severe, or profound, depending on how loud sound has to be before it is perceived. Figure 2-10 shows the ranges of each of these types of hearing impairment. When you look at Figure 2-11, you will see that the low frequencies are in the severe loss range, and high frequencies are in the profound range. Now, if you understand what we mean when we say that this audiogram shows "a severe to profound sensorineural hearing impairment" — you've got it!

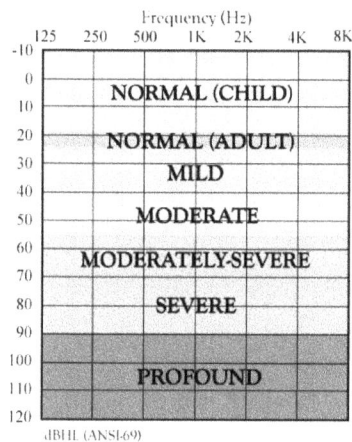

Figure 2-10 Ranges of hearing impairment

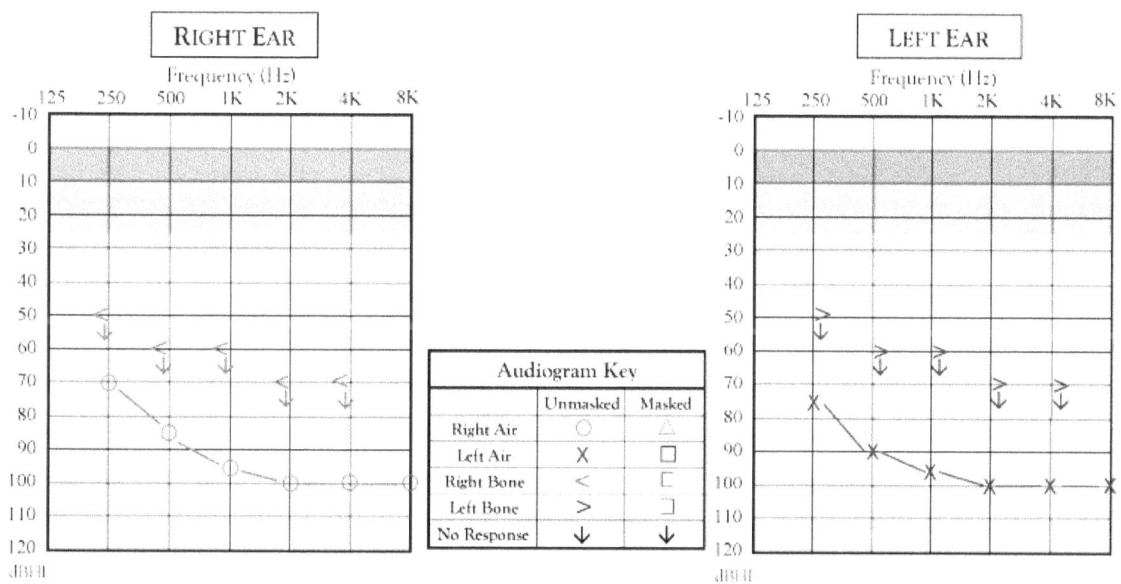

Figure 2-11 Severe to profound sensorineural hearing impairment

For an interactive and animated description of an audiogram, please follow this link:

http://www.letthemhear.org/hearing/implants.php# and click on "View the animations to learn about audiograms."

Key Takeaways

1. Several professionals, each with a unique set of skills and knowledge, are involved in the process of defining the exact level of hearing impairment and its cause.

2. You are the coach of your team. Take the time to put together the best team of professionals possible.

3. It is extremely important to find a pediatric audiologist and an ear physician as soon as possible. These are the two key players who will help you answer the earliest questions.

4. The first questions, which you must answer as soon as possible, are: Is there a hearing loss present? And if so, what is the type and level?

5. Seek out other families in your area who have been in your shoes. They can offer their experience and advice.

6. Hearing testing can be completed at any age, but for very young children, testing requires specific equipment and highly trained personnel that are not available at all facilities. It is important to select a facility that has this equipment and personnel.

7. Depending on the age and developmental skill level of the individual, subjective and/or objective testing may be performed to determine the exact type and level of hearing impairment. It may require several visits to paint a clear picture of your child's hearing impairment.

8. The two most common types of hearing impairment are sensorineural and conductive. Sensorineural hearing impairment exists when sound reaches the cochlea but has trouble reaching the brain. Conductive hearing impairment exists when either a permanent or temporary blockage prevents sound from reaching the cochlea.

9. Hearing impairment is measured in units called decibels, often abbreviated as dB, and levels can range from normal to profound.

10. The audiogram is the graph that will paint a picture of your child's hearing impairment. Learn how to read and understand this.

Chapter 3

Other Issues Associated with Hearing Impairment

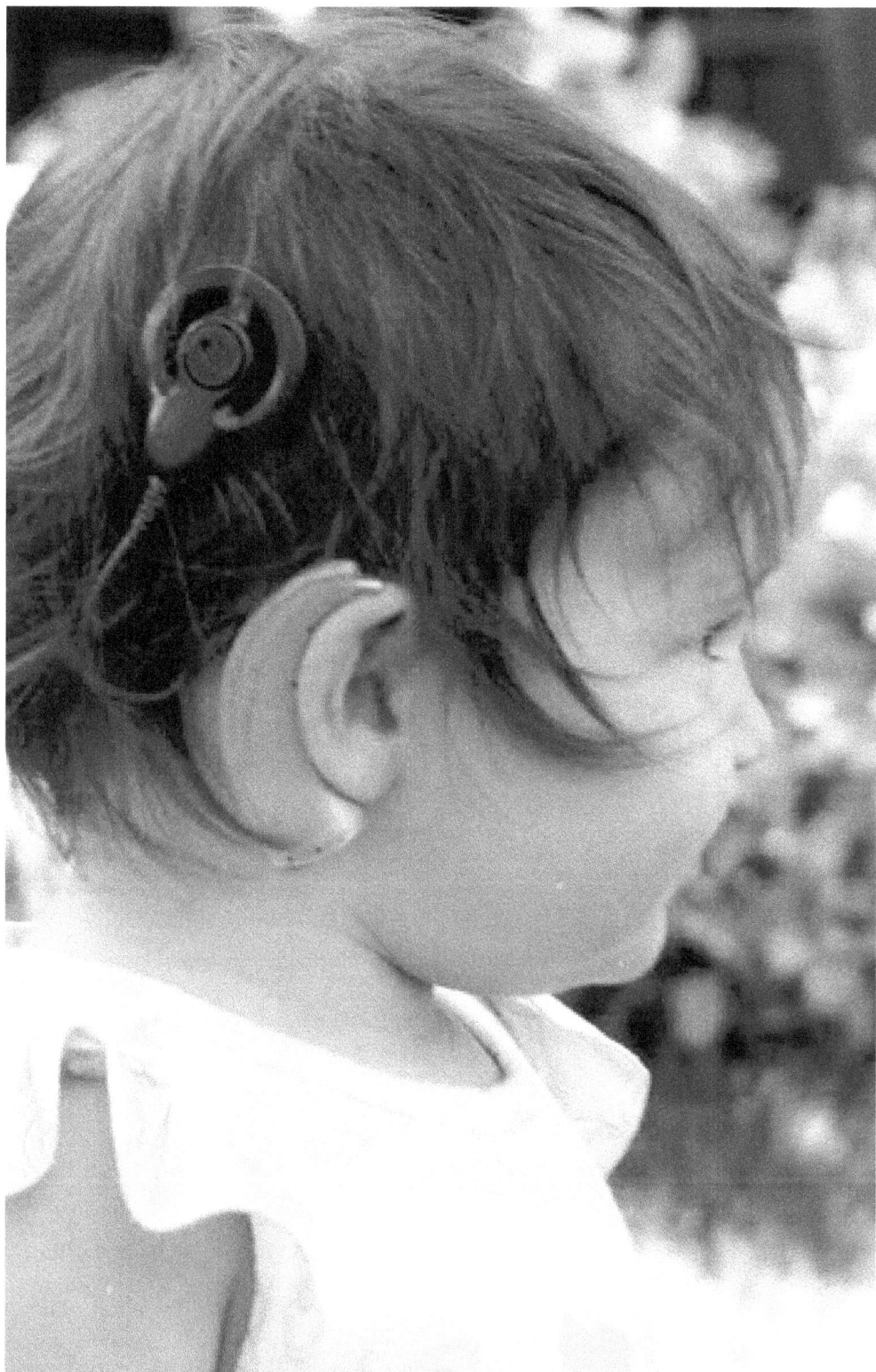

Introduction

Now that we have identified the hearing problem and outlined your support team, we need to discuss other issues your child may need to address associated with hearing impairment. The following chapter discusses other medical conditions that could arise along with a hearing impairment, as well as examinations that should be performed. A staggering 40 percent of infants with hearing impairment have some other medically significant condition. Sometimes these other health problems combined with the hearing impairment result in a syndrome, which is a grouping of medical conditions that commonly arise together. Other times, the medical condition, such as asthma or astigmatism, might be completely separate from the hearing impairment.

There are more than 100 different sources of hearing impairment. Many of the congenital sources are genetic, and many of the more common genetic sources now can be conclusively identified through a simple blood test. The area of genetics and genetic diagnosis has exploded over the past decade and will continue to do so over the next several decades. A team that keeps up-to-date with these developments is best.

Depending on the results of genetic testing, a thorough physical exam, and review of family history, other medical follow-up tests may be recommended.

Examinations and Preventive Care

Eye Examinations

It is important for any child with hearing impairment to have ophthalmology examinations conducted regularly as part of follow-up care. Hearing-impaired children rely heavily on their vision in order to read lips (now referred to as "speech reading") to augment their communication abilities. Even a slight vision loss or distortion may adversely affect a hearing-impaired child's ability to communicate. Another major concern is Usher's syndrome, which is a common source of hearing impairment and is strongly associated with retinitis pigmentosa. Usher's syndrome frequently leaves individuals both hearing-impaired and blind by adulthood, although the visual problems associated with some types of Usher's syndrome frequently don't present themselves until the teenage years or even later.

Radiological Examinations

Many radiological examinations are used to rule out or diagnose issues commonly associated with hearing impairment. Almost all hearing-impaired children will receive a CT scan shortly after the diagnosis is made. CT scans allow otologists to investigate for cochlear abnormalities known as Mondini malformations, common cavities, or enlarged vestibular aqueducts. A magnetic resonance imaging (MRI) scan may also be separately ordered in some cases.

Other Organ/Systems Evaluation

Hearing impairment can be a symptom of several syndromes, each of which has many different components. Therefore, in a thorough pediatric hearing impairment work-up, tests for thyroid function and kidney function (including urinalysis, blood tests, and kidney imaging), back or neck X-rays, heart tests, and other immunological or infectious blood testing may also be indicated. As the child gets older, other testing may be ordered, including growth hormone testing and computerized dynamic posturography or electronystagmography to analyze the vestibular (balance) system. Children who continue to struggle in school more than their audiograms might predict may receive additional testing for attention deficit disorder, dyslexia, or auditory processing function.

Vaccinations

It is especially important that all children with hearing impairments receive all meningitis and pneumonia vaccinations as soon as possible. Children with hearing impairments, either with or without cochlear implants, are at higher risk of contracting meningitis than the general population. In addition, the Prevnar vaccination for pneumonia has the side effect of reducing ear infections by approximately 30 percent.

Ear Infections

Ear infections are a common childhood illness. Of course, adults get them too, but because the eustachian tube function is poorer in children, they are more likely to develop ear infections. Most of the time, occasional ear infections are not cause for significant alarm. However, they present a more complex challenge for hearing-impaired individuals for two reasons:

1. The fluid associated with ear infections can cause temporary additional hearing impairment (conductive) on top of the existing hearing impairment.
2. If the ear is actively draining, as sometimes occurs with an ear infection, hearing devices cannot be worn.

Otitis Media

Middle ear infection (otitis media) often occurs after a cold or infection of the upper airways. The eustachian tubes drain fluid from the ears to the back of the throat, and these tubes can become swollen and blocked during a cold. When this happens, the fluid in the ears is unable to drain and collects in the middle ear space. This fluid is now susceptible to germs, which can cause a bacterial infection.

The middle ear is a pocket of air behind the tympanic membrane, or eardrum. The eustachian tubes run from the middle ear to the back of the nose. When you need to equalize pressure on both sides of the eardrum—during takeoff in an airplane, for example—you can swallow or yawn, which forces the tube open and allows the air on either side to equalize. During an ear infection, pressure from excess fluid builds up and presses on the eardrum, causing pain, and the tube cannot be opened up to either drain the fluid or equalize the pressure.

The typical symptoms of otitis media are ear pain, fever, decrease in hearing, and occasionally dizziness, which, if severe, can lead to vomiting. If there is drainage from the ear, it could be caused by a perforation, or hole, in the eardrum. This is commonly referred to as the eardrum "bursting." If this occurs, like a ruptured appendix, it will generally be accompanied by a decrease in pain because the pressure on the eardrum has been relieved. In this case, even though the child feels better, he or she should be seen by a doctor as soon as possible.

Glue Ear

Glue ear is another common condition that mainly affects children between the ages of two and five. It is characterized by a sticky glue-like substance that collects in the middle ear behind the eardrum. It may cause a temporary loss of hearing, but if left untreated, it could cause permanent hearing impairment.

The medical terms for glue ear are "otitis media with effusion," "secretory otitis media," and "chronic secretory otitis media." We can see from these terms that it is a condition of the middle ear, with a slightly different mechanism than otitis media.

The middle ear, as well as being attached to the eustachian tubes, has a lining similar to that of your lungs. Air passes through this lining to the bloodstream, but if the eustachian tubes become blocked, a vacuum is formed in the middle ear and the lining can become inflamed. Once inflamed, the lining begins secreting a fluid, which thickens and leads to glue ear.

Just like otitis media, glue ear is a common after-effect of colds. It can also be caused by allergies or other irritants such as dust or cigarette smoke in the air. It is quite often seen in children with cleft palates due to poor eustachian tube function.

Glue ear affects hearing, and in very young children it can lead to delays in speech and language development. In older children, it can cause balance problems, as well as a decrease in hearing ability. Turning the TV louder, asking for words to be repeated, frequently saying "what" or "huh," and unusual clumsiness may be indications of glue ear.

Glue ear can last a long time, but most children eventually recover from it naturally. Antibiotics or decongestants may be prescribed to lessen the fluid buildup. The condition should be followed for several months to see if any other complications develop.

Ear Infection Treatment

Antibiotics are the standard treatment once an ear infection has been diagnosed. Although the underlying respiratory infection that may have caused the ear infection is viral, the ear infection itself will be bacterial in nature. The type of antibiotic used will depend on what antibiotics were successful for the child's previous ear infections and whether the patient has any antibiotic allergies. Antibiotics may include oral medications or topical antibiotics in the form of ear drops. It is extremely important to follow the full duration of the medication or the infection may not clear up completely. This will result in it returning, possibly in a form that is more resistant to the type of antibiotics that were originally prescribed.

An over-the-counter decongestant such as pseudoephedrine (often sold under the brand name Sudafed) can assist in reducing the fluid associated with ear infections and glue ear. Discomfort and fever can be treated with acetaminophen (Tylenol) or ibuprofen; however, these symptoms usually diminish quickly once the antibiotics begin to work.

If the patient does not respond to antibiotics or has two infections in a six-month period, then more aggressive treatment is needed. Glue ear and recurring ear infections that do not respond to antibiotics may be surgically treated via a procedure called myringotomy, or with the placement of a temporary pressure equalization (PE) tube in the eardrum.

Myringotomy is a simple surgical procedure. A hole is made in the eardrum so that fluid, which cannot drain through the blocked eustachian tubes, can instead drain through the hole in the eardrum. This hole will close up on its own in approximately six weeks. This option is frequently chosen when a patient needs to fly on an airplane but has significant fluid behind the eardrum, preventing them from doing so.

If the hole needs to be kept open for more than six weeks, then a tube, sometimes called a PE or pressure equalization tube, can be inserted through the eardrum to keep the hole open. The tube also lets air into the middle ear, allowing the ear to function normally.

Precautions need to be taken when a patient has a hole in the eardrum. These precautions include wearing ear plugs when swimming or placing the head under water in the bath tub. Diving should be avoided.

Most PE tubes are considered temporary, especially in children. As the eardrum grows, the tube will be pushed out, generally within a year of insertion. Many times the patient will have recovered adequately enough that the tubes need not be replaced. However, if the pattern of ear infections reoccurs, tube placement can be repeated. Multiple repeated tube placements can scar the eardrum and result in permanent hearing impairment. Typically, PE tubes are placed in the operating room under general anesthesia. The procedure generally lasts less than twenty minutes. However, for older children and adults, and especially for those who have already had one set of PE tubes placed, it may be possible to insert a replacement set of PE tubes in the office under a local anesthetic.

Ear Infection Prevention

Preventing an ear infection from occurring is much better than having to treat one after it occurs. The following simple steps may be useful in reducing the number of ear infections experienced by a patient who suffers from chronic ear infections.

Keep the Ear Dry

"Swimmer's Ear" drops can be used after the ear is exposed to water (either from swimming or bathing) to help reduce moisture, which creates a breeding ground for the bacteria that cause ear infections. These can be purchased over the counter at most drugstores.

Get a Pneumococcal Vaccination

A vaccine is now available that may protect children against ear infections. Although it was originally developed as a pneumonia vaccine, the bacteria that it targets are also responsible for approximately one-third of ear infections and other respiratory infections. It can also protect against meningitis.

The pneumococcal vaccine, known as Prevnar or PCV7, is now recommended for all children up to the age of two. Older children who are susceptible to ear infections can also benefit from the vaccine. It is especially useful in reducing the number of infections for patients who don't respond well to antibiotics.

Reduce Allergic Reactions and Upper Respiratory Infections

Because so many ear infections start out as fluid buildup due to colds or allergies, any of the standard steps taken to reduce colds is also likely to reduce the number of ear infections the patient experiences. Standard techniques for reducing colds include more frequent hand washing, avoiding group settings (such as playgrounds) with a large number of children who may be spreading germs during the cold season, and taking over-the-counter supplements such as vitamin C or Echinacea, which have been linked to reductions in colds. Improving your overall immune system health by reducing stress and getting an adequate amount of sleep may also have a positive impact on the number of colds and ear infections.

To reduce allergic reactions, an individual must first identify the item or items that he or she is allergic to. This can be done through skin testing or a blood test, or by eliminating common allergens and watching to see if the allergy symptoms improve. Once identified, allergies can be treated by eliminating exposure to the items that trigger allergies; using over-the-counter and prescription drugs, including nasal sprays; getting allergy shots; and using sublingual (under the tongue) immunotherapy.

Tonsillectomy/Adenoidectomy/Mastoidectomy

In extreme cases, chronic ear infections may be made worse by congenital malformations such as cleft palate, oversized tonsils or adenoids, or an infection in the mastoid bone. In these cases, it may be necessary to surgically remove the tonsils and/or adenoids. In the case of mastoid bone infection, a procedure called mastoidectomy may be performed to remove the underlying cause of the recurring ear infections. These surgeries, while extremely common thirty years ago, are less common today because of the invention of better antibiotics and other less-invasive treatments. They should be considered treatments of last resort.

Otitis Externa and Earwax Buildup

Otitis externa is an ear infection that occurs in the ear canal itself, on the outside of the eardrum. Otitis externa can have several contributing factors, including earwax buildup and impacted hairs.

Earwax, also known as cerumen, is not really wax, but debris that builds up in the ear canal over time. Some of the debris comes from the shedding of skin cells from the canal wall, but the debris can also include blood or pus from previous ear infections. Earwax production typically increases over time; adults produce substantially more earwax than do children.

Individuals who are born without ear canals (atresia) and have ear canals created through a surgical procedure known as atresia repair suffer from greater earwax accumulation problems. This is because the skin that is grafted to create the ear canal wall sheds cells at a much higher rate than would normal ear canal wall skin. It is also well documented that in times of significant stress, especially illness or surgery, earwax production can drastically increase.

Certain types of ear molds worn in the canal with hearing aids are also associated with higher levels of earwax buildup. Molds that fully block the ear canal are associated with higher levels of earwax accumulation. Vented ear molds or open-fit ear molds, which allow more air to circulate in the ear canal, are associated with lower levels of earwax accumulation. The style of mold used with hearing aids depends on the individual's level of hearing impairment. Your child's audiologist will recommend an appropriate style of ear mold.

Earwax accumulation can cause temporary conductive hearing impairments of up to 40 decibels. Wax pushed up against the eardrum will prevent the eardrum from vibrating, as well as blocking the sound from getting to the cochlea. Earwax accumulation can also create a moist environment, contributing to otitis externa infections. However, you should never attempt to remove earwax from your child's ear. Cotton swabs should not be used to remove earwax, as they can damage the eardrum and even dislocate the middle ear bones if pushed too deep into the ear canal. Instead, you should visit an ENT, who will use a microscope and remove the wax using either suction or forceps.

Finally, since soft earwax is easier to remove than hard earwax, it is important to take steps to keep the earwax soft, such as using drops of olive oil or hydrogen peroxide rinses. This can make for a more comfortable earwax removal experience for your child.

Perforated Eardrum

An eardrum perforation is a tear or other opening in the delicate tympanic membrane, also known as the eardrum. Sometimes this is referred to as a burst or ruptured eardrum. Perforations can be single, or there may be multiple perforations in various locations on the eardrum. The location and number of perforations influence the ability of the eardrum to heal and also affect how great the resulting hearing impairment is. Any eardrum abnormality will increase the risk of infections and perforations, which can result in temporary or even permanent hearing impairment.

Perforated eardrums have many causes. They are frequently the result of infection. Various types of trauma to the ear can also result in a hole in the eardrum and possible hearing impairment; an example would be striking the ear on the water's surface in a fall while wakeboarding. Injury to the eardrum can also occur when such objects as cotton swabs, bobby pins, or other objects are used in an attempt to remove wax from the ear. A very loud noise, such as an explosion, can also cause a perforation or other injury to the ear. Less common causes of perforations include a fractured skull, a lightning strike, or a hot spark or slag entering the ear while welding. Changes in air pressure, called barotrauma, can occasionally cause eardrum perforation. This may occur when flying or scuba diving with a severe cold.

The usual symptoms of an eardrum perforation are either discharge from the ear (otorrhea), earache (otalgia), or a change in hearing. Bleeding or pus from the ear may indicate the presence of a perforation. A subtler symptom may be that the ear just doesn't feel right.

In severe trauma to the ear, as seen in skull fractures, in addition to eardrum perforation, there may also be damage to the three middle ear bones, or ossicles. In these cases, the loss of hearing may be severe and is often associated with ringing of the ears, also called tinnitus.

Perforated eardrums are diagnosed by a thorough examination of the ears by a physician; this exam may be carried out by a pediatrician or family practitioner. A small instrument called an otoscope may be used, or the exam may be more exactly accomplished by use of an operating microscope by specially trained physicians. A hearing test (audiogram) can also help in making the diagnosis.

Some conditions that lead to perforated eardrums can be treated or prevented. Common sense tips include:

- Do not ignore ear infection symptoms. All suspected ear infections should be assessed and treated as promptly as possible, and any prescribed antibiotics should be taken until completion.
- Never try to remove an object that is lodged in your ear canal.
- Do not use objects such as cotton swabs, bobby pins, or paper clips in your ears in an attempt to clean them.
- Do your best to avoid contact with persons who have colds or flu-like illnesses.
- Make certain that children are current with their immunizations, as recommended by their pediatricians. In particular, the Prevnar vaccination is estimated to reduce the number of ear infections by 10 to 20 percent in children with recurrent ear infections.

Many eardrum perforations heal on their own. This is particularly true of smaller perforations located toward the center of the eardrum. Larger perforations may require a surgical procedure called a tympanoplasty. This is a form of microsurgery in which tissue is removed from another part of the body, usually around the ear, and attached (grafted) to the area of the eardrum that is perforated. In some cases, the tympanoplasty procedure may be done along with other surgeries, including repair of the three small bones of hearing in the middle ear, if they are involved. The surgery is usually performed on an outpatient basis. Tympanoplasty surgeries have a high rate of success. In most cases, the perforation is closed permanently and hearing is improved.

Sensory Processing Disorders

Sensory processing disorders are a complex set of disorders of the brain that affect developing children. These disorders are mostly seen in hearing-impaired individuals (and also some normal hearing individuals) due to the abnormal processing of sound at the brain level. The lack of normal sound through the brain produces a poor maturation and dysfunction of the system. Children with sensory processing disorders misinterpret everyday sensory information, including information from the five basic senses (touch, sound, sight, smell, taste), as well as movement-related sensory input from the vestibular system, and/or the positional sense, known as proprioception. This misinterpretation can result in a child feeling overwhelmed with sensory information. These children may seek out intense sensory experiences, which can lead to behavioral problems. These disorders are also associated with problems with gross and fine motor skills. Therapy can help mitigate these symptoms, but far too many children are not properly diagnosed with sensory processing disorders and as a result do not receive this therapy.

Originally, the phrase "sensory integration dysfunction" was used to describe abnormal social, emotional, motor, and functional patterns of behavior that were related to poor processing of sensory stimuli. In fact, the theory, which was proposed by Dr. A. Jean Ayres, who pioneered research in this area, is still referred to as "sensory integration theory." However, as research in this area better defined specific types of disorders, the diagnostic terminology evolved. The phrase "sensory processing disorder" is now used to define a diagnostic category that contains three separate types of sensory disorders: sensory modulation disorder, sensory-based motor disorder, and sensory discrimination disorder.

Sensory modulation disorder is diagnosed when there is either an over- or under-response to sensory stimuli or seeking sensory stimulation. Individuals with sensory modulation disorder exhibit patterns of fearful and/or anxious reactions, negative and/or stubborn behaviors, and self-absorbed behaviors, in which the individual is either difficult to engage or creates or actively seeks sensation. Sensory modulation problems can include:

- Sensory registration problems, characterized by the failure of the affected individual to notice stimuli that are ordinarily obvious to others.

- Sensory defensiveness, characterized by over-responsiveness in one or more sensory systems.

- Gravitational insecurity, characterized by the tendency to react negatively and fearfully to movement experiences, particularly those involving a change in head position and movement backward or upward through space.

Sensory-based motor disorder is diagnosed when the affected individual has disorganized motor functions that are the result of incorrect processing of sensory information and feedback. This exhibits itself primarily as coordination problems and fine and/or gross motor skills issues.

Sensory discrimination disorder involves challenges with sensory discrimination or postural control and/or dyspraxia, which is a disorder that affects motor skill development. It can result in inattentiveness, disorganization, and poor school performance.

Children who are suspected to have a sensory processing dysfunction are generally tested somewhere between the ages of four and a half and eight years. The test most frequently used to assess these children is the Sensory Integration and Praxis Test. Once a child is diagnosed, an occupational therapist will typically be sought out to initiate a therapy program. The occupational therapist can also provide valuable input on environmental accommodations that parents and school staff can use to enhance the child's function at home, at school, and in the community. These accommodations may include selecting soft, tag-free clothing, avoiding fluorescent lighting, and providing ear plugs for difficult situations, such as fire drills.

Auditory Processing Disorder

Auditory processing disorder may appear alone, or it may appear in a child who is hearing-impaired. When auditory processing disorder and hearing impairment are combined, a child may appear to be more hearing-impaired than the audiogram would otherwise indicate. Some of the symptoms of auditory processing disorder include:

- Difficulty paying attention to and remembering verbal information

- Problems following multistep directions

- Poor listening skills

- Requiring additional time to process information

- Low academic performance

- Behavior problems

- Language difficulties such as confusing syllable sequences, and problems developing vocabulary and understanding language

- Difficulty with reading, comprehension, spelling, and vocabulary

Therapies and equipment that are available to assist children with auditory processing disorders in developing compensatory skills include:

- FM systems, discussed in more detail in Chapter 5

- Improvements in classroom acoustics, discussed in more detail in Chapter 7

- Language-building exercises, which can increase the ability to learn new words and increase a child's language base

- Auditory memory enhancement, a procedure that reduces detailed information to a more basic representation

- Informal auditory training techniques, which can be used by teachers and therapists to address specific difficulties

Attention-Deficit Hyperactivity Disorder

Attention-deficit hyperactivity disorder (ADHD) has many symptoms in common with hearing impairment. Many situations have been reported in the scientific literature in which children are diagnosed with ADHD (or, in the past, ADD) and do not respond to medication. Later, these children are found to have undiagnosed hearing impairments. However, it is quite possible for a child with a hearing impairment to also have ADHD, which requires additional specific treatment. For these children, it is especially important to have a skilled diagnosis by a doctor who is capable of distinguishing between behaviors attributable to the hearing impairment and behaviors attributable to ADHD.

The main confusion arises from the fact that several of the main symptoms of ADHD overlap with symptoms of hearing impairment. Children with ADHD, hearing impairment, or both may present with symptoms of inattention, problems with task completion, disruptive behavior, noncompliance, speech and language problems, or a need for frequent repetition of information. In an article titled "Attention Deficit and Hyperactivity Disorder: What Is Currently Known and Its Significance for ENT Specialists," the authors specifically recommended that all ENTs consider hearing impairment as a potential differential diagnosis for any child presenting at the ENT clinic with an ADHD diagnosis and unknown hearing status.

Furthermore, in "Diagnosis and Management of Attention Deficit Hyperactivity Disorder in Primary Care for School Age Children and Adolescents," the U.S. government noted that "50% of children with ADHD are likely to have communication/interaction problems that manifest themselves as social skills deficits" and suggested that all children with ADHD diagnoses be screened for hearing impairment.

Hyperacusis

Hyperacusis is characterized by oversensitivity to certain sounds. While hyperacusis is more common in adults, it is also known to occur in children. Hyperacusis can be either congenital or acquired. In acquired hyperacusis, some of the causes that are more likely to occur in children include noise trauma and chronic ear infections. Hyperacusis in children is also associated with autism spectrum disorders such as Asperger's syndrome. In general, any child may cry or fuss when exposed to loud noises. However, if children respond negatively to everyday sound levels, including clanking dishes, barking dogs, traffic noises, or common sounds such as running motors, by running away, covering their ears, or screaming loudly, they should be evaluated to see if hyperacusis is present.

Key Takeaways

1. Otitis media and glue ear are common childhood illnesses that create a more complex challenge for individuals with hearing loss because they can cause

additional, temporary hearing impairment. If the ear infection is active, hearing devices should not be worn.

2. Ear infection symptoms should not be ignored. These include pain, fever, and decreased hearing. Make an appointment to see your ear, nose, and throat physician if an ear infection is suspected.

3. Antibiotics are the first course of treatment for ear infections and may be in the form of oral medication or ear drops. It is extremely important to follow the entire course of antibiotics through to the end.

4. Glue ear and recurring ear infections require more aggressive treatment, such as myringotomy (where a hole is created in the eardrum to allow for fluid drainage) or PE tube placement (where a small tube is placed in the hole to keep it open for a longer period of time).

5. It is important to keep your child's ear dry if he or she has a hole in the eardrum. Use swim plugs while swimming, and avoid placing the child's head underwater during bath time.

6. Simple steps such as keeping the ear dry and having your child vaccinated against the pneumococcal virus may reduce the number of ear infections a child experiences.

7. Earwax is a buildup of debris in the ear canal and should be monitored by your child's ear, nose, and throat physician and audiologist. You should never stick anything in the ear in an attempt to remove earwax.

8. A perforated eardrum, also known as a burst or ruptured eardrum, can be caused by an ear infection or trauma to the ear, and can result in additional hearing impairment, which may be temporary or permanent.

9. Sensory processing disorders and auditory processing disorders may be present in children with hearing impairment and present additional challenges when managing these children.

10. Symptoms of hearing impairment, auditory processing disorders, and ADHD sometimes overlap, making the differential diagnosis of these disorders difficult. It is important to find a skilled doctor who is familiar with the diagnosis of these conditions.

Chapter 4

Which Language Destination Is Right for My Child?

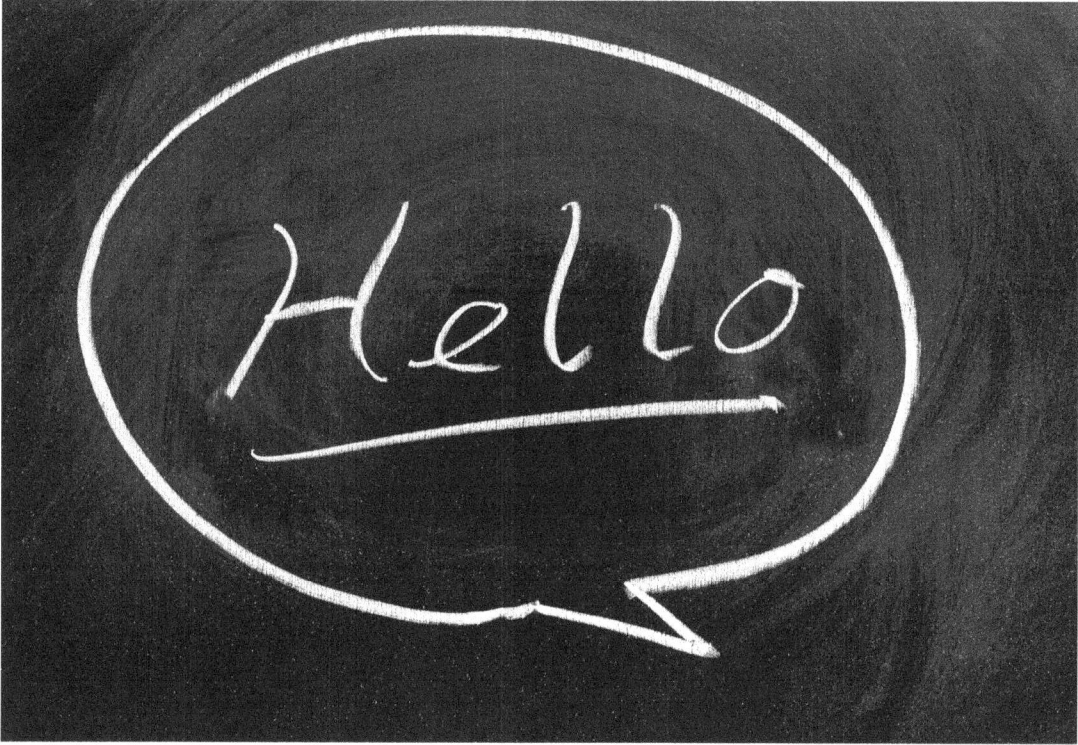

Introduction

Creating a comprehensive treatment plan for your child with hearing impairment is a little bit like figuring out travel plans for a multiday drive across the country; unless you know the destination first, chances are you aren't going to end up where you want to be at the end.

In the case of hearing impairment, the destination is the mode of communication that your child will master. The available language destinations are speaking, signing, or some combination of the two. The initial choice of language destination for your child will drive many important decisions, including which types of doctors and specialists you see, which types of treatment you consider, and what types of therapy are most appropriate.

Regardless of your child's language destination, it is important to remember that you, the parent, are the coach of your child's hearing impairment team. You will decide which doctors to see, what types of follow-up medical and language evaluations to perform, and what types of treatment or devices to select. You will also make the final decisions about ongoing maintenance and upgrading of those devices. In the case of conflicting advice, it is you who will decide which advice to follow.

Communication Modalities

A communication modality is the method one person uses to communicate with another. For hearing people, there is frequently just one communication modality, and that is speech. However, for individuals with hearing impairment, there are many communications options, each with its own plusses and minuses.

Auditory-Oral

The auditory-oral approach is a communication modality in which children with hearing impairment learn to use whatever hearing they have, in combination with the contextual cues of speech/lip reading, to understand and use spoken language. The goal is to give the hearing-impaired child the necessary spoken language skills to be able to successfully function in a mainstream education environment and to function independently in the hearing world.

The auditory-oral communications modality is frequently the choice of cochlear implant recipients. If the purpose of undergoing surgery to receive a cochlear implant is to restore hearing to normal or near-normal levels, then it follows that the communication modality that makes the most use of that hearing is the most likely choice. If the family's desired outcome is spoken communication, the child's auditory brain centers must be accessed and developed.

The auditory-oral approach facilitates the development of reading and writing skills, because proficiency in the English language is critical to developing good reading ability. Competence in reading is critical to learning in all academic areas. Small self-contained classrooms coupled with daily individualized instruction and therapy provide the intense early intervention needed in this approach. Teachers in these programs are highly trained and provide spoken language instruction throughout the day in all classroom activities. This is full-time therapy and education.

The auditory-oral modality is also a communication option for individuals who do not have cochlear implants but use hearing aids instead. This approach may also be used with individuals who are cochlear implant candidates but choose not to receive a cochlear implant. This is because the modality's emphasis is on teaching the children to maximize the hearing they have; good hearing is not a requirement to use this modality.

Several scientific papers support the validity of the auditory-oral communications modality, including:

1. Moog, Geers, Tobin and other researchers focused on <u>aural/oral habilitation with cochlear implants.</u>
2. <u>Existing Evidence that Supports the Rationale for Auditory-Verbal Practice...</u>
3. <u>Cochlear implants in adults and children.</u> (NIH Consensus Development Panel on Cochlear Implants in Adults and Children)

Auditory-Verbal

The auditory-oral and auditory-verbal communications modalities have several similarities:

- Both approaches intend to promote listening, thinking, speaking, and communication for children with all degrees of hearing impairment.

- Both approaches emphasize brain access through residual (remaining) hearing aided by the most appropriate technology—hearing aids, cochlear implants, FM systems, etc.—to establish listening, thinking, speaking, and communicating.

- Both approaches require that hearing is emphasized and utilized before vision.

However, there are subtle but meaningful differences between the two modalities. In the auditory-verbal communications modality, families follow a specific set of guiding principles to enable their child who is hearing-impaired to learn to listen to and process spoken language. Although families who participate in auditory-oral programs may utilize strategies and techniques of the auditory-verbal approach, an auditory-verbal intervention program embraces all guiding principles.

The most noticeable practical difference between the two modalities may be that traditional auditory-oral programs rely on therapists and teachers as models, and children who are hearing-impaired may receive instruction or therapy in groups, sometimes in special schools or classrooms. The auditory-verbal approach, in contrast, emphasizes integrating the child into mainstream settings as much as possible. The goal is to educate the child in the least restrictive environment (LRE) with the highest expectations, and the mainstream classroom serves as the default in this approach.

Declared principles of auditory-verbal practice include:

- To detect hearing impairment as early as possible through screening programs, ideally in place in the newborn nursery and throughout childhood.

- To pursue prompt and vigorous medical and audiologic management, including selection, modification, and maintenance of appropriate hearing aids, cochlear implants, or other sensory aids.

- To guide, counsel, and support parents and caregivers as the primary models for spoken language through listening, and to help them understand the impact that hearing impairment has on the entire family.

- To help children integrate listening into their development of communication and social skills.

- To support children's auditory-verbal development through one-on-one teaching.

- To help children monitor their own voices and the voices of others in order to enhance the intelligibility of their spoken language.

- To use developmental patterns of listening, language, speech, and cognition to stimulate natural communication.

- To continuously assess and evaluate children's development in the above areas and, through diagnostic intervention, modify the program when needed.

- To provide support services to facilitate children's educational and social inclusion in regular education classes.

American Sign Language

American Sign Language, or ASL, is a complete, signed language with its own grammar, word order, and expressions. It differs from spoken language in that it uses hand movements combined with facial expressions and postures of the body. It is the primary language of the majority of Deaf individuals in North America and is associated with the Deaf culture, which has its own customs and beliefs. No one signed language is universal; different sign languages are used in different countries. Many individuals believe that the use of sign language with young children, whether they are hearing-impaired or have normal hearing, can promote early communication.

Signed Exact English

Signed Exact English, or SEE, is a system of manual communication that strives to be an exact signed representation of English vocabulary and grammar. SEE takes much of its vocabulary of signs from ASL. However, SEE frequently modifies the hand shapes used in the signs borrowed from ASL to incorporate the hand shape used for the first letter of the English word that the SEE sign is meant to represent. SEE has also added many new signs, especially signs for grammatical concepts and articles that are not part of ASL. This strict faithfulness to spoken English constructs means that using SEE for communication is slower than spoken language or ASL.

Unlike ASL, SEE is not considered a language on its own. Rather, it is a manual recoding of an existing spoken language—namely, English. Thus, there is some dispute about whether foreign language credit ought to be given for SEE proficiency or classes, as is commonly done now with ASL.

SEE mirrors English grammar, including full use of articles and prepositions. Some people think this feature assists hearing-impaired children who may have difficulty learning the correct usage of these parts of the English language. Also, SEE is easy for people who already speak English, such as the hearing parents of hearing-impaired children, to master quickly.

Cued Speech

A speech reader is one who uses speech reading to understand speech. According to Galluadet University's website, speech reading is the ability to perceive speech by watching the movements of a speaker's mouth, by observing other visual cues, such as facial expressions and gestures, and using the context of the message and the situation. Only a small percentage of speech is visible to a speech reader. About 70 percent of speech cannot be seen on the lips. For example, hearing individuals can hear the difference between the voiced words "pat" and "bat," but if you make the motions associated with these words in the mirror and do not voice them, the mouth motion looks almost identical. Good speech readers will be able to figure out by sentence context if the word was "pat" or "bat," but even the best speech reader will miss a lot of these phrases.

Cued Speech is a system of communication that makes traditionally spoken languages accessible by using a small number of hand shapes (representing consonants) in different locations near the mouth (representing vowels), as a supplement to speech reading. Using the above example, Cued Speech attempts to remove some of the uncertainty from duplicated mouth motions representing multiple words by combining a hand motion and placement on the face with the mouth motion, which visually indicates to the speech reader whether the speaker said "pat" or bat" without requiring understanding of the context.

Cued Speech may look similar to other forms of signing communication such as ASL or SEE, but it is not. Cued Speech is a manual communications mode that represents English words at the phonological level. Cued Speech has been adapted to more than 60 languages and dialects, including some tonal languages, where the inclination and movement of the hand is used in addition to hand shape and placement of the hand to indicate the appropriate tone.

Total Communication

Total Communication, or TC, is an approach to educating hearing-impaired children that utilizes several modes of communication, including signed, oral, auditory, and written and visual aids, depending on the particular needs and abilities of the child. One of the major intents of Total Communication is to act as a middle ground between the opposite ends of the hearing-impairment education spectrum—auditory-oral, which focuses exclusively on speech, and signing, which focuses exclusively on a manual-based language.

The philosophy behind Total Communication is that the communication method should fit the child, rather than forcing the child to use a communication method that he or she may find uncomfortable. In the Total Communication world, any form and any combination of communication forms is acceptable. This includes any form of sign language, voice, finger spelling, lip reading, amplification, writing, gestures, and visual imagery (pictures). The anything-goes approach fostered by Total Communication creates an environment that encourages hearing-impaired children to communicate in any form they choose, rather than restricting communication to a single path, such as signing only or auditory-oral only.

Studies are mixed on the effect that Total Communication has on language development of hearing-impaired children in the long term. Some researchers express concern that use of the Total Communication model results in hearing-impaired children failing to become fluent in either a signed language or a spoken language because of the imperfect use of both, and the acceptability of resorting to other options (such as writing and gestures) when both fail. Other researchers favor Total Communication as a model that ensures that hearing-impaired children have access to some means of communication all the time.

One thing that is certain is that Total Communication, as a language model, lacks any standards or organizing body to ensure its consistent implementation in schools for the hearing-impaired around the country. Another issue is that, although individualization is at the heart of the Total Communication philosophy, teachers are limited in how many modes they can use at one time. This makes it impossible for one teacher to meet all the communication needs that are present in a group setting.

Bilingual/Bicultural

Bilingual-bicultural, or BiBi, education of the hearing-impaired is based on the principle that American Sign Language (ASL) is the language most completely accessible to hearing-impaired children. However, BiBi also recognizes that these hearing-impaired children will need to live and succeed in the hearing world. In addition, BiBi education recognizes and respects that the vast majority of hearing-impaired children come from hearing families, with family members who use speech as their primary form of communication.

For these reasons, the BiBi philosophy supports the use of ASL for all instruction, with a strong commitment to written English literacy. Another key component to the BiBi approach is to actively teach children to understand and accept the differences between the hearing and hearing-impaired communities.

Does My Child Have a Language Delay?

The National Institutes of Health has identified a comprehensive list of milestones to assist in determining whether a child has normal speech and language development. It is important to keep in mind that every child is different and may develop at a faster or slower pace. This list serves as a general guideline to monitor your child's speech and language development.

Speech and Language Milestones: Birth to Five Months

1. Reacts to loud sounds

2. Turns head toward a sound source

3. Watches your face when you speak

4. Vocalizes pleasure and displeasure sounds (laughs, giggles, cries, or fusses)

5. Makes noise when talked to

Speech and Language Milestones: Six to Eleven Months

1. Understands "no-no"

2. Babbles (says "ba-ba-ba" or "ma-ma-ma")

3. Tries to communicate by actions or gestures

4. Tries to repeat your sounds

Speech and Language Milestones: Twelve to Seventeen Months

1. Attends to a book or toy for about two minutes

2. Follows simple directions accompanied by gestures

3. Answers simple questions nonverbally

4. Points to objects, pictures, and family members

5. Says two to three words to label a person or object (pronunciation may not be clear)

6. Tries to imitate simple words

Speech and Language Milestones: Eighteen to Twenty-Three Months

1. Enjoys being read to

2. Follows simple commands without gestures

3. Points to simple body parts such as "nose"

4. Understands simple verbs such as "eat," "sleep"

5. Correctly pronounces most vowels and n, m, p, h, especially in the beginning of syllables and short words; also begins to use other speech sounds

6. Says eight to ten words (pronunciation may still be unclear)

7. Asks for common foods by name

Speech and Language Milestones: Two to Three Years

1. Knows about fifty words at twenty-four months

2. Knows some spatial concepts such as "in," "on"

3. Knows pronouns such as "you," "me," "her"

4. Knows descriptive words such as "big," "happy"

5. Says around forty words at twenty-four months

6. Speech is becoming more accurate but may still leave off ending sounds; strangers may not be able to understand much of what is said

7. Answers simple questions

8. Begins to use more pronouns such as "you," "I"

9. Speaks in two- to three-word phrases

10. Uses question inflection to ask for something (e.g., "My ball?")

11. Begins to use plurals such as "shoes" or "socks" and regular past tense verbs such as "jumped"

Speech and Language Milestones: Three to Four Years

1. Groups objects such as foods, clothes, etc.

2. Identifies colors

3. Uses most speech sounds, but may distort some of the more difficult sounds, such as *l, r, s, sh, ch, y, v, z, th*; these sounds may not be fully mastered until age seven or eight

4. Uses consonants in the beginning, middle, and ends of words; some of the more difficult consonants may be distorted, but are attempted

5. Strangers are able to understand much of what is said

6. Able to describe the use of objects such as a fork, a car, etc.

7. Has fun with language; enjoys poems and recognizes language absurdities such as, "Is that an elephant on your head?"

8. Expresses ideas and feelings rather than just talking about the world around him or her

9. Uses verbs that end in "ing," such as "walking," "talking"

10. Answers simple questions such as, "What do you do when you are hungry?"

11. Repeats sentences

Speech and Language Milestones: Four to Five Years

1. Understands spatial concepts such as "behind," "next to"

2. Understands complex questions

3. Speech is understandable but makes mistakes pronouncing long, difficult, or complex words such as "hippopotamus"

4. Says about 200 to 300 different words

5. Uses some irregular past tense verbs such as "ran," "fell"

6. Describes how to do things such as painting a picture

7. Defines words

8. Lists items that belong in a category such as animals, vehicles, etc.

9. Answers "why" questions

Speech and Language Milestones: Five Years

1. Understands more than 2,000 words

2. Understands time sequences (what happened first, second, third, etc.)

3. Carries out a series of three directions

4. Understands rhyming

5. Engages in conversation

6. Sentences can be eight or more words in length

7. Uses compound and complex sentences

8. Describes objects

9. Uses imagination to create stories

Key Takeaways

1. A communication modality is the way in which one person communicates with another. There are many different communication options, and as the parent and "coach" of your child's team, it is up to you to choose your child's method of communication.

2. In the auditory-oral approach, children with hearing impairment are taught to use the hearing they do have in combination with speech/lip reading in order to understand and use spoken language.

3. The auditory-oral approach is often used by cochlear implant recipients.

4. The auditory-verbal approach is similar to auditory-oral in that both promote the use of spoken language through listening; however, families who choose the auditory-verbal approach follow a strict set of guidelines to enable their children to communicate using spoken language.

5. American Sign Language (ASL) is a complex form of manual communication in which hands, limbs, head, facial expression, and body language are used to communicate. ASL is not related to spoken English, and features an entirely different grammar and vocabulary. Linguistically, it is a complete and fully realized language in its own right.

6. Signed Exact English (SEE) is a manual form of communication that mirrors the vocabulary and grammar of the English language.

7. The Total Communication (TC) approach follows an anything-goes philosophy. TC encourages children to communicate in any form they choose, whether that be signing, spoken language, writing, gestures, etc.

8. Cued speech is a system of hand gestures and placement of these gestures near the mouth that allow the speechreader to differentiate between words that would otherwise by indistinguishable through speechreading alone.

9. The bilingual/bicultural (BiBi) approach centers around ASL as the primary form of communication, with a strong commitment to developing written English literacy. The bicultural aspect comes from the education of these children on the differences between the hearing and Deaf communities.

10. It is important to monitor your child's speech and language development to ensure that he or she is reaching appropriate milestones. Refer to the list developed by the National Institutes of Health outlined in this section.

Chapter 5

Treatment Options: How to Enable Your Child to Hear

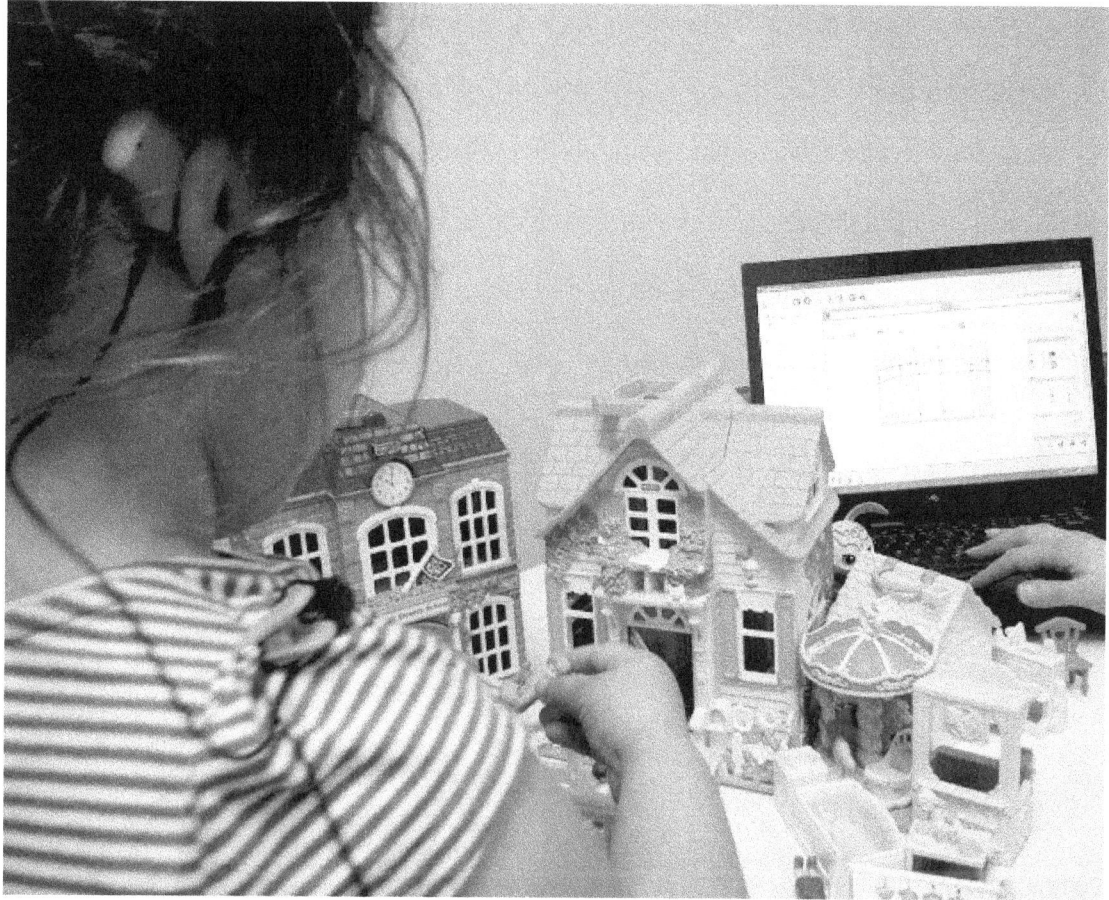

Introduction

There are many avenues of treatment for hearing loss. Not every option will be appropriate for your child or for his or her level or type of hearing loss. It is important to discuss the options with your audiologist and ear physician. More than one option may be appropriate, and you may try multiple options before settling on the most beneficial one. Some options are more expensive than others, but for right now, try to focus on what will be best for your child. In a later section, we will discuss funding options.

Hearing Aids

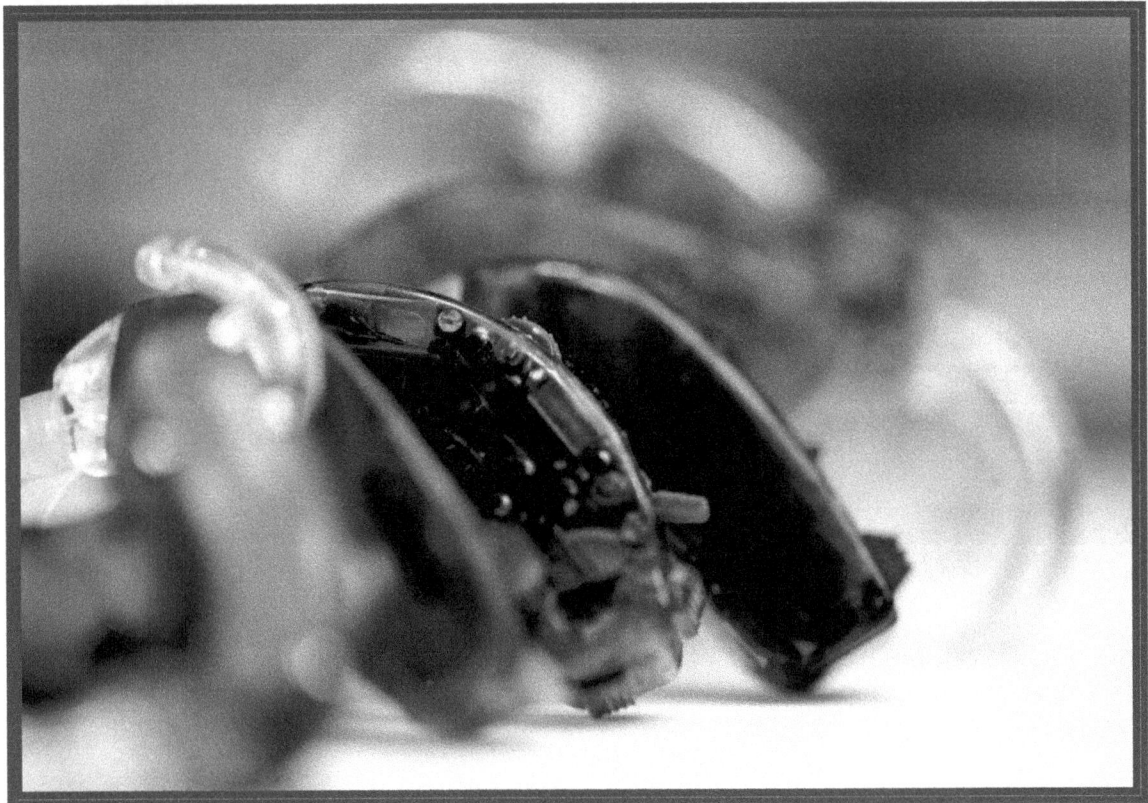

Electronic hearing aids have been with us for more than fifty years. Their initial basic design principle is still in use today: take a sound and make it louder, so it can be more easily heard. Of course, there have been improvements over the past fifty years. Hearing aids pretty much used to be one-size-fits-all, with no ability to customize based on the age of the patient or the level of hearing impairment. Because of the miniaturization of electronics, hearing aids now come in several configurations, including:

- Behind the ear (BTE)

- In the ear (ITE)

- Completely in canal (CIC)

- Contralateral routing of sound (CROS)

- Bone conduction hearing aids

Additionally, different models of hearing aids are now made to fit different levels of losses. For example, power hearing aids are used only for people with severe to profound losses, while an open-fit hearing aid model might be used to fit a mild or moderate hearing impairment.

Analog vs. Digital Hearing Aids

Traditional hearing aids use analog circuitry; in other words, the sound signal is processed entirely in the analog domain, which is how humans normally perceive sound.

In the past decade, a new type of hearing aid has appeared on the market: the digital hearing aid. These devices allow sound to be processed in various ways. The processing can help to improve the clarity of desired sounds (i.e., speech) while eliminating background noise or other unwanted sounds.

To get a better idea of the advantages or disadvantages of each type of hearing aid, let's look a bit at how they have evolved over the years. The earliest transistor hearing aids were simple amplifiers; they made *everything* louder. In quiet environments, this helped a person with hearing impairment to better understand speech or television or radio. In noisy environments, however, the hearing aid was often a disadvantage, because the background noise would simply be too distracting.

The next step in the development of the hearing aid was to make it adjustable. The audiologist would measure the patient's hearing impairment and send the specifications to a laboratory, where a customized hearing aid would then be built. The device could be individually tailored for specific hearing problems using frequency analysis and filters. This way, the entire spectrum of sound was not amplified, but only the particular frequencies that the patient needed.

This was a big improvement, but it didn't address the problem of hearing needs in different noise environments. Thus, the programmable hearing aid was developed; this was designed to be user-adjustable for different situations. The device could be adjusted by a remote control, allowing the patient to apply different filters and settings according to hearing need. Programmable devices were a step forward, but there were still limitations in the number of different settings available to the user.

Digital hearing aids first came on the market in the late 1980s. Their use of digital signal processing allowed a much more flexible approach to adjusting frequency amplification. Unfortunately, the earliest digital models were quite bulky and had a short battery life, so they were relatively unsuccessful on the market. By the late 1990s, the technology had improved to the point where digital hearing aids were a practical alternative. Their high cost was offset by the improved signal processing offered over analog devices.

The advantages of digital hearing aids lie completely in their ability to process sound. The audiologist has many options available to tailor the device to the patient's needs. Individual frequency bands can be amplified or reduced, and the shape of the frequency band can be set.

Generally speaking, the digital hearing aid has five components: the microphone, the analog-to-digital converter, the processing unit, the digital-to-analog converter, and the receiver. Sound is picked up by the microphone and then converted into digital information. The processing unit changes the sound according to what kind of hearing impairment the patient experiences. After the processing, the sound is converted back to analog and fed into the receiver so the user can hear the sound.

The processing unit is what gives digital hearing aids an edge over their analog counterparts. Digital signal processing allows certain parts of the sounds—bands of frequencies— to be amplified, while at the same time reducing unwanted frequencies. Digital hearing aids can do this with much more precision than analog. Thus, vocal frequencies can be focused on, while removing distracting background ambient noise.

Feedback, the high-pitched squealing noise that often occurs when the sound being amplified is picked up by the hearing aid microphone and reamplified, can be reduced or eliminated with digital hearing aids. The digital hearing aid monitors for feedback, and prevents it by applying a suppression mechanism.

A few special features are found on digital hearing aids. The directional microphone allows you to focus on sounds in front of you, while eliminating sounds coming from behind. This can be great in crowd situations where you are trying to talk with one person but there is a lot of noise all around you.

Today, digital hearing aids can automatically switch between directional and omnidirectional (allowing amplification of all sounds around you). In quiet situations, you will generally want to hear sound from different directions (omnidirectional). For example, at home, if someone speaks to you from the side, you would not hear them when the microphone is set to directional.

Newer digital hearing aids have the ability to switch settings for different situations. These changes in settings occur automatically, as the hearing aids select an optimal amplification function depending on whether the environment is noisy or quiet, or whether you are listening to music or talking to someone. Newer hearing aid features include integration with Bluetooth devices such as cell phones.

Digital hearing aids are more expensive than analog, but as the technology continues to improve and manufacturing procedures become more commonplace, the price will surely decrease. We are seeing greater miniaturization in the computer field, and this will spill over into providing smaller and more effective hearing aids in the future.

Hearing Aid Routine for Children

If your child has a mild or greater hearing impairment, it is likely that hearing aids will be recommended, either as a permanent solution, if the aids result in hearing levels that allow your child to gain meaningful auditory input, or as a trial solution, to see if your child receives adequate benefit from hearing aids before considering cochlear implantation.

Starting a regular schedule for hearing aid use can be hard. However, it is important to establish a routine with respect to hearing aid use with your child as soon as possible, and it is best to keep trying every day. Some infants accept hearing aid use quite easily. Other infants may not like having something in their ears, just as some infants don't accept wearing hats or shoes immediately. Some infants may be fine about wearing hearing aids when they are quite young, but may begin to pull them out and stick them in their mouths as they get older and more curious about the world around them.

If your child doesn't readily accept the hearing aids, or begins a phase of pulling them out, you can try to build up his or her tolerance for wearing them over time. The eventual goal is to have your child wearing the hearing aids for the majority of his or her waking hours. However, this is not always possible. The most important times to wear hearing aids are when there is direct contact and communication between your infant and either you or one of your child's therapists.

As children get older and the behavior of the "terrible twos" begins to kick in, sometimes the children use their hearing aids as a battle in the power struggle with their parents. It is important that you, as the parent, are in charge of hearing aid use. You are in charge of putting the hearing aids in and taking them out. Even if your child is pulling the hearing aids out frequently, you can put the hearing aids right back in, and set a time goal for keeping them in. Your audiologist, early intervention specialist, or therapists can give you more ideas to help with keeping the hearing aids in. Discussing this issue with families who have faced similar problems, in either in-person or online support groups, may also result in creative solutions that have your child keeping the hearing aids in more regularly and for longer periods of time. Do not be afraid to share your problems or questions with these groups of people.

Morning Hearing Aid Routine

Follow this routine every morning:

- Check the batteries.
- Check the ear mold(s) for any debris, such as wax or dirt, blocking the opening.

- Listen to the sound produced by the hearing aid using a listening scope. If your child wears power aids, be sure to use a filter when listening so that you don't damage your own hearing.

- Insert the hearing aid. You may need Oto-Ease or a similar lubricant.

If the hearing aids squeal after they've been inserted correctly, it is likely due to a poor-fitting ear mold. This frequently occurs as children grow rapidly and the ear molds become too small. When this happens, you will need to visit your audiologist and have new ear impressions taken. These will be sent to the manufacturer, and a new set of ear molds will be created. In the earlier years, this can occur as frequently as once every two to three months. A lotion called OtoFerm may help temporarily eliminate squealing until the new ear molds can be obtained, which generally takes at least two weeks. If the OtoFerm is not sufficient to reduce the feedback, special pads called Comply Wraps can be wrapped around the canal of the ear mold to improve the fit and stop the feedback until new ear molds can be made. These products can be obtained from your audiologist.

Hearing aids should be worn during all waking hours, except any time they may get wet—for example, when swimming or bathing.

Bedtime Hearing Aid Routine

Follow this routine each evening at bedtime:

- Remove the hearing aids.

- Gently remove the ear molds, trying not to pull on the tubing. Inspect them for any dirt or debris. Remove any earwax from the ear mold with a wax loop, provided by your audiologist.

- Place the hearing aids in the dry aid kit. (Do this every night, and immediately if the hearing aids get wet from water or sweat.)

- The battery doors should remain open while in the dry aid kit.

- Note the color of the crystals and reactivate them if necessary in the microwave or the oven.

General Hearing Aid Routine

In addition to the daily morning and bedtime routines, there are a few other routines to follow:

- Remove the ear molds from the hearing aids and gently wash them once a week, using warm water and mild dish soap without additives. Rinse thoroughly. You can do this more often if you notice wax buildup more than weekly.

- After washing, dry the ear molds on a paper towel overnight. Use the air blower to clear the tubing, and then place them in the dry aid kit.

- Moisture and humidity are extremely damaging to hearing aids. If you live in an area with particularly bad humidity, a dry aid kit or a "Dry and Store" is essential to keep the electronics as dry as possible.

Keeping Hearing Aids in Place

Keeping hearing aids in place for infants and toddlers can be a challenge. There are many simple solutions available to help reduce this problem.

It helps to begin by understanding why the hearing aids are coming out. They may come out on their own, or the children may pull them out due to curiosity or irritation. The first thing is to determine whether there is an audiologically significant reason behind why they are pulling the hearing aids out, or the aids are falling out. Electronic problems such as static, amplification cutting out, poorly fit ear molds, or hearing aid programs that are not properly aiding the child's loss (because they are too loud or too soft) might be the source of the problem. Your child's audiologist can help you investigate these issues.

It is important that the smaller pediatric tone hooks are used for infant and children's hearing aids. When the larger hooks are used, the bulk of the hearing aid electronics are less likely to sit snugly behind the ear, and the weight swinging forward may dislodge the ear mold.

Clips can be used to attach hearing aids to a child's clothing. These devices keep the hearing aids connected to the child's clothing so that they don't go too far even if they do come out. Some name brands for these devices include Huggie Aids, Critter Clips, Kid Clips, Ear Gear, and SafeNSound security straps. Some hearing aids come with the ability to run dental floss or fishing line through small holes and then attach that thread to the clothing. Even devices intended to keep pacifiers or eyeglasses from getting lost are low-cost solutions that will help keep hearing aids from getting lost.

For children who do not have adhesive allergies, toupee or wig tape can also be used to help hold the hearing aids in place behind the ears. This tape needs to be changed frequently and monitored for irritation. Tie-on caps (such as Hanna Andersson pilot caps) can also be used to keep children from pulling hearing aids out while still allowing sound to be picked up by the hearing aids' directional microphones.

Finally, brightly colored ear molds, stickers on the hearing aids, or other hearing aid markers such as nail polish can be visual clues to help find hearing aids when all else has failed and the hearing aid is lost on a sidewalk, or in tan bark or sand on a playground.

Hearing Aid Insurance

One of the most important issues concerning parents about hearing aids coming out is that hearing aids have a "trifecta" combination of bad factors: they are small, expensive, and extremely easy to misplace. Because of this, it is especially important that parents maintain an active loss/damage insurance policy for their infant's hearing devices. This is available through the following sources:

1. Initial hearing aid purchases frequently come with a two-year repair warranty and a one-year loss and damage warranty. Usually, the loss replacement portion of the warranty can only be used one time, and the damage portion of the warranty does not include normal wear and tear repairs.

2. Extended warranties can sometimes be obtained for free at the time the aids are purchased if you use a credit card that automatically offers this option for electronics. This is a little-used but extremely valuable option that may double the initial warranty offered by the manufacturer.

3. Once the initial warranty runs out, hearing aid manufacturers generally offer extended warranties that can be purchased to continue the coverage.

4. Separate insurance specific for hearing aids can be purchased from companies like Ear Services Corporation. Premiums are generally based on a percentage of the replacement cost of the devices.

5. Riders may be available on homeowner's or renter's insurance covering the loss, theft, or destruction of hearing aids, just as you would add a rider to a policy for expensive computer equipment or jewelry.

Treatment for Single-Sided Deafness

Traditionally, physicians and audiologists have been taught that if one ear is normal, then auditory, speech, and language function and development will be normal. We now know this long-held belief is absolutely incorrect. The basics of auditory function dictate that the brain takes an auditory signal, then analyzes it to give us the sensation we know as hearing. In noisy and low-volume environments, the brain has to have a signal from both ears to do its job correctly.

Untreated single-sided hearing impairment in children produces several functional and developmental problems. It is fair to say, based on up-to-date research, that the more difficult the listening situation, the more dysfunctional single-sided hearing becomes. For example, a child with unilateral hearing impairment may function relatively normally at home in a quiet environment, interacting with one known speaker who knows about the hearing impairment. That same child may have extreme difficulty in a noisy classroom. Even if teachers, parents, and professionals think the child is doing "just fine" with hearing only on one side, it is well-documented that untreated single-sided hearing impairment has a significant potential impact on adult earning potential.[5] Children with single-sided hearing impairment may have difficulty with sound localization, hearing in noise, managing cognitive load, and overcoming the head shadow effect. Each of these is discussed more in-depth below.

---

[5] U.S. Census Bureau, 1997. Survey of Income and Program Participation tables.

Kochkin, S. The Impact of Untreated Hearing impairment on Household Income, August 2005, Better Hearing Institute, Alexandria, VA, viewable at
http://www.betterhearing.org/pdfs/MarkeTrak7_ImpactUntreatedHLIncome.pdf

Sound Localization

We have all had the experience of being in a very noisy restaurant and trying to listen to someone across the table from us. That is a very practical example of what someone with hearing only on one side experiences during a significant portion of the day. When children have functional hearing in only one ear, that same feeling occurs with very low levels of background noise.

Auditory input from two ears provides the listener with the ability to localize sound. When a sound comes at us from any angle, the brain measures the difference in time it takes for the sound to reach each ear. For example, a sound coming from the right will register in the right ear before it does in the left. This interaural (between ears) time difference is very small, but when two ears hear a sound at slightly different times, the source of the sound can be localized and the listener can turn to it, if desired. Just like the loss of vision in one eye eliminates depth perception, the loss of hearing in one ear eliminates the hearing equivalent, which is sound localization. Imagine yourself on the playground, and someone is calling your name, and you can hear him or her but cannot tell where the sound is coming from. That is what hearing with a single ear produces. We believe this is one reason why children with single-sided hearing impairment have almost twice the rate of injury of those with normal hearing in both ears.[6]

---

[6] Mann, J.R., Zhou, Li, McKee, M., McDermott, S. "Children with Hearing Impairment and Increased Risk of Injury." *Annals of Family Medicine* (2007): 5:528-533.

Hearing in Noise

Another benefit of auditory input from two ears is the ability to better understand speech in noisy environments. Every day we select out the speech we want to listen to from a sea of noise. To go back to our analogy above, all of us have had trouble hearing another person speaking to us in very noisy situations, like a restaurant or party. The brain, not the ear, is responsible for our ability to listen selectively. For this system to function correctly, hearing from two ears is essential. Without two hearing ears, a child will have difficulty hearing speech in the presence of even small amounts of background noise. Every brain is different in its ability to perform this task, and testing can be done to evaluate this ability. On some occasions, the brain has trouble with this task even when two normally hearing ears are present, as in the case of auditory neuropathy.

Managing Cognitive Load

Understanding speech in noisy environments while conducting tasks is difficult even for people with normal levels of hearing. The louder the background noise, the longer it takes the individual to complete a task, the more mistakes are made in performing that task, and the more speech the individual misses. This concept is called "cognitive load" and can represent a subtle but constant problem for school-aged children attempting to understand what a teacher is saying while taking notes in a noisy classroom.

Head Shadow Effect

A person with normal hearing and brain function can preferentially listen with one ear instead of the other through the use of the head shadow effect. The head shadow effect is the brain's ability to turn up one ear (the ear toward the sound signal one wants to hear) and turn down one ear (the ear that is away from the signal one wants to hear) using the head as a block or shadow to block out unwanted noise. Imagine you are walking down a sidewalk with noisy traffic to one side and a friend talking to you from the other. Your brain will preferentially listen to your friend, and will effectively turn down the volume for the ear on the other side to improve understanding. Now imagine a teacher walking around a noisy classroom, and imagine what happens when the teacher walks to the side with hearing impairment or turns to write on the blackboard. With that image, you can understand how two ears are preferable to a single ear in the classroom and other life situations.

Children with Single-Sided Deafness Should Be Aided

The brain's ability to hear in noise is not present at birth; it develops over time during the first ten to twelve years of life. This system only develops fully when both ears are providing auditory input to the brain. Waiting until late in this process to provide hearing in both ears does not make sense from a developmental standpoint.

For this reason and the reasons listed above, it should be all otologists' medical objective to return hearing to both ears, if at all possible, and as early as possible. As stated above, in the past, physicians were taught that one ear is good enough, and thus many do not recommend treatment of single-sided deafness. Physicians who are poorly informed about the current research do not see a problem in delaying treatment of single-sided hearing impairment during the very critical period of development of the auditory system during the first few years of life. Unfortunately, this delay can create permanent and irreversible harm to the child whose hearing impairment goes untreated.

A professional who is able to give treatment options and chances of success must assess individual situations. These options may change over time. For example, surgery to perform atresia repair may be the right choice if a CT scan shows a high chance of success at the appropriate age. Additionally, a bone anchored prosthetic device worn on a soft-band may be the right treatment to stimulate the ear and hearing nerve from a few weeks of age until this CT evaluation for surgery is possible.

Surgically Implanted Auditory Prosthetics

In addition to hearing aids that are completely removable, surgically implanted auditory prosthetics are available to assist individuals with hearing impairment. Devices on the market today include:

- Bone-anchored prosthetic devices

- Middle ear implantable hearing aids such as the Vibrant Soundbridge and Otologic MET

- Cochlear implants

The difference between surgically implanted auditory prosthetics and completely removable hearing devices is important. Hearing aids enhance hearing through amplification, meaning that they take sound and make it louder. Surgically implanted auditory prosthetics function differently. Rather than amplifying sound, they take sound and find a different mechanism to get that sound to the brain without amplification. While this differentiation may not seem crucial to the operation of the device (because the end result in each case is improved hearing), it is extremely important from a financial perspective. Most private and public insurers in the United States do not provide coverage for devices to improve hearing (i.e., hearing aids), but most do cover auditory prosthetics, and in several states, coverage is mandated by law.

Bone-Anchored Prosthetic Devices

Bone-anchored prosthetic devices are manufactured by Cochlear (the Baha) and Oticon (the Ponto). Each device consists of three parts:

1. A titanium screw, which is implanted into the skull

2. A titanium abutment, which is attached to the screw

3. An external sound processor that snaps onto the titanium abutment

For young children, the external sound processor can be worn on a headband (frequently referred to as a "softband") until the child's skull has become thick enough for the titanium components to be implanted, typically around five or six years of age. Implantation provides an average of 9 decibels better gain and between 14 and 20 percent higher speech recognition scores. This is because when implanted, the sound processor no longer has to vibrate through skin and hair to do its job.

Bone-anchored prosthetic device implantation surgery takes less than ninety minutes and is relatively minor. The titanium screw must "osseointegrate"—that is, have time to become tightly bound to the bone in the skull—before the external sound processor can be worn. Some ongoing care and follow-up is required after the surgery to keep the skin around the abutment healthy.

Who Benefits from Bone-Anchored Prosthetic Devices?

Three groups of people can benefit from bone-anchored prosthetic device implantation:

1. Those with purely conductive hearing impairment, regardless of whether it is unilateral or bilateral.

2. Those with a profound sensorineural hearing impairment on one side and normal hearing on the other side.

3. Those with a mixed hearing impairment, regardless of whether it is unilateral or bilateral, as long as the bone conduction thresholds on the worse of the two sides are 25 decibels or better in the speech frequencies (approximately 300 to 5,000 Hz).

Bone-anchored prosthetic device implantation is generally reserved for individuals who have failed more conservative approaches to treatment and cannot benefit from traditional hearing aids. Under FDA criteria in the United States, children must be five years old before the bone-anchored prosthetic device can be implanted. In Canada and Europe, implantation frequently occurs at 18 months of age. Therefore, the FDA limit is not a practical limit, but a limit used by insurers to avoid paying for this device for younger children in the United States.

How Do Bone-Anchored Prosthetic Devices Work?

All bone-anchored prosthetic devices use direct bone conduction. The device is placed on the hearing-impaired side behind the ear, and it transfers sound through bone conduction using the skull. In the case of individuals with conductive loss, these skull vibrations bypass whatever is causing the conductive loss and stimulate both functioning cochleas and auditory nerves. In the case of individuals with single-sided hearing impairment (i.e. profound sensorineural hearing impairment on one side only), the skull vibrations stimulate the cochlea and auditory nerve of the ear with normal hearing.

The bone-anchored prosthetic device provides the opportunity for individuals to hear and understand sounds from both sides of the head, where previously the head shadow effect totally blocked certain sounds. This ultimately results in the sensation of hearing sound from the hearing-impaired side.

Middle Ear Implantable Hearing Devices

Middle ear implantable hearing devices correct hearing impairment through the direct surgical implantation of a device into the middle ear. Because there is no component of a middle ear implantable hearing device in the canal, these devices are particularly good for individuals who have issues with chronic infections, feedback, occlusion, or canal abnormalities that make wearing a traditional hearing aid impossible.

Globally, three different middle ear implantable hearing devices are currently available: the Vibrant Soundbridge, manufactured by Med-el; the MET, manufactured by Otologics; and the DACS, manufactured by Cochlear. We will not go into detail regarding these devices, as none of these devices is currently approved in the United States for use in children; however, some of them have been successfully used in children in clinical trials.

Cochlear Implants

How Do Cochlear Implants Function?

Cochlear implants are implantable electronic devices that can bring hearing to profoundly hearing-impaired individuals. A cochlear implant bypasses the outer and middle ear functions and sends electronic sound stimulation directly to the auditory nerve, then to the brain, where it is interpreted as sound.

An operation is required to surgically implant the internal portion of the device, known as the electrode. A patient must also wear an external device that looks like a behind-the-ear hearing aid with an attached circular coil. Environmental sound is received by the external electronics behind the ear and transmitted across the skin via the circular coil to the internal device. The internal device makes use of a surgically implanted electrode inserted inside the cochlea that releases electrical energy (instead of the usual vibrational energy utilized by the cochlea) to stimulate the hearing nerve. In essence, a cochlear implant bypasses the damaged nerve cells, called hair cells, in the cochlea and stimulates the hearing nerve directly.

Here is how a cochlear implant works. Once implanted, the speech processor microphone picks up sound. For children under the age of three, the speech processor is generally worn in a belt on the body. For children over the age of three and adults, the speech processor is generally worn in a behind-the-ear style.

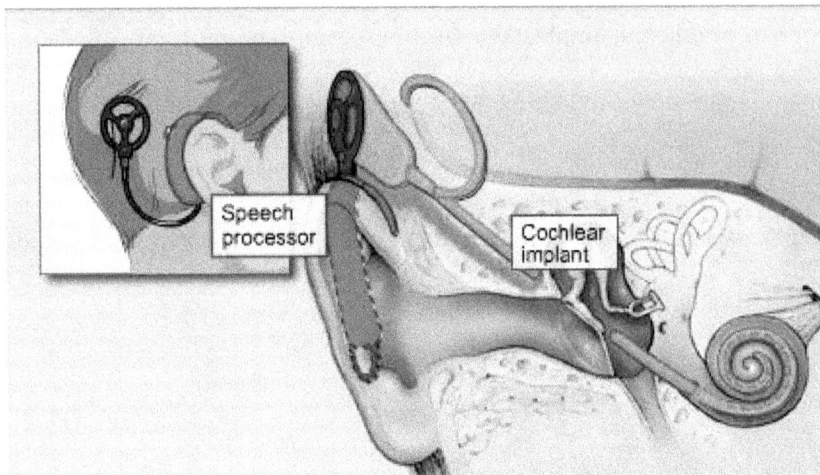

The speech processor (item 1 in the image below) analyzes the sound and digitizes it into coded signals, then sends those coded signals to the transmitting coil (item 3 in the image below).

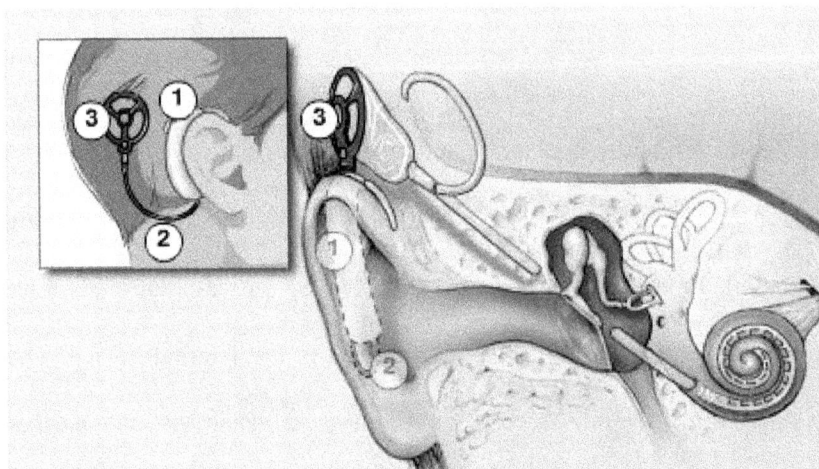

The transmitting coil then further sends the signals to the cochlear implant receiver/stimulator (item 4 in the image below) under the skin, which then delivers the appropriate amount of electrical energy to the array of electrodes inside the cochlea (item 5 in the image below).

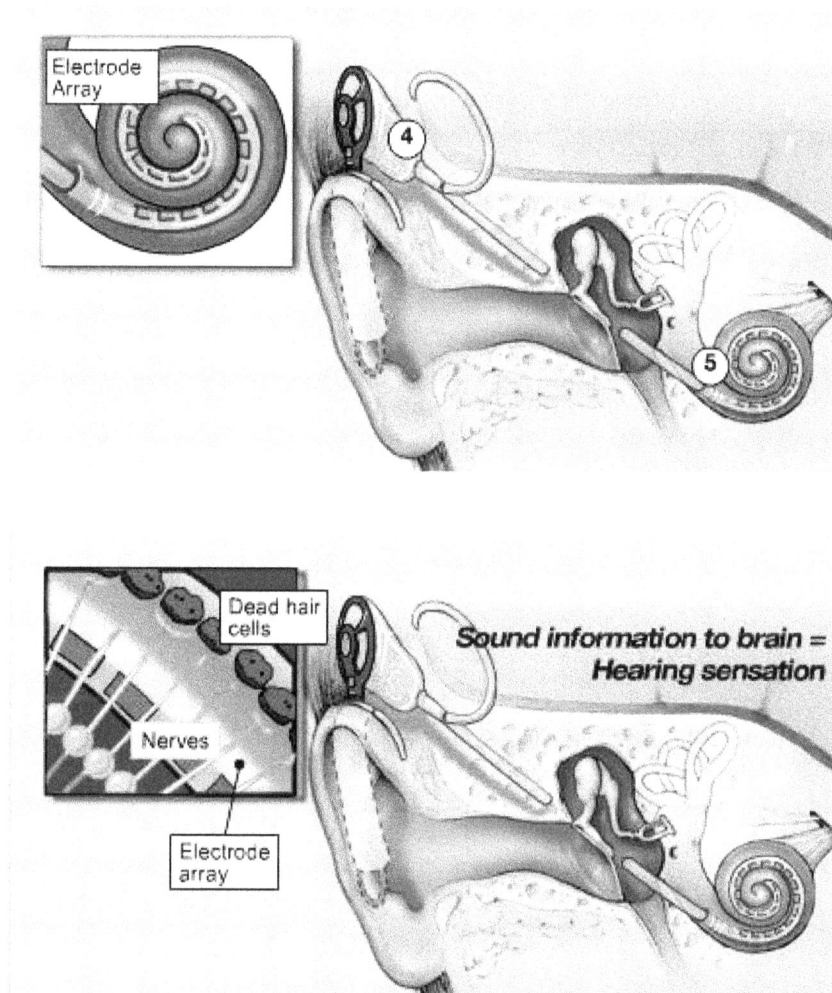

It is these electrodes that stimulate the auditory nerve, which then sends the electrical sound information through the auditory system to the brain, which generates the sensation of hearing.

Who Benefits from Cochlear Implants?

Cochlear implants have the best results with respect to the ability to hear and understand speech in two categories of patients: previously hearing individuals who have lost their hearing (known as "postlingual deafness") and children born deaf (known as "prelingual deafness") when implanted early in life.

Postlingual deafness occurs when deafness comes on after a period of hearing, which has allowed development of speech and language. Many causes of postlingual deafness are possible, including meningitis, exposure to medications toxic to the inner ear, trauma, and progressive genetic causes, among others. Postlingually deaf patients do well with cochlear implants because their ears have heard during the critical period of development in the first five years of life, allowing the brain to develop the neural connections of sound processing. Those nerve pathways often remain when the nerve cell receptors are damaged through the process that resulted in the hearing impairment.

The pathways can atrophy, or weaken, somewhat when not used for many years, but they will be reactivated when a cochlear implant sends signals through the neural pathways again. Consequently, the signal can be perceived as very close to what normal speech sounds like. When a postlingually deafened individual is asked, "What does it sound like?" after receiving a cochlear implant and undergoing the appropriate rehabilitation and therapy, they generally will say something like, "It's not 100 percent normal but it's close," or, "It's about 80 to 90 percent of normal speech for me."

Keep in mind that the brain is used to receiving electrical signals from a normal inner ear. As the software and electrical processing of cochlear implants become better at simulating the way the hearing nerve usually codes speech signals, the sound gets better and better, and closer and closer to normal. Eventually, with a lot of work and experimentation, scientists may be able to produce hearing that is better than normal.

Fortunately, cochlear implants are built so that future software upgrades can be loaded into the external device, allowing for improved performance over the years without requiring extra surgical procedures. This is very important, as this process is happening at a remarkable rate of speed. Twenty-five years ago, patients were told to only expect sound awareness, with little to no chance of understanding speech. Today, we expect about 85 percent of postlingually deafened patients who receive cochlear implants to be able to use the telephone and have significant open set speech recognition.

Prelingual deafness is present congenitally (at birth) or just after birth, before the brain has a chance to develop the neural pathways used to handle sound. This is a very important concept. If the brain does not receive sound input during the time when it would normally develop the neural pathways used for hearing, speech, and language, then the possibility of future development is lost and cannot be regained later. Five years of age is too late. Most of the language development burst occurs during the first two to three years of life. Lifelong effects on brain function occur. Once you understand this principle, you will understand how absolutely critical it is that hearing impairment is addressed as early as possible.

A cochlear implant inserted early in this time period will allow normal development of the brain's auditory pathways. The age of implantation has steadily dropped over the past twenty-five years. Initially, cochlear implants were only approved for adults. When they were approved for children, at first, the youngest children were two and a half years, then two years, then eighteen months. Now twelve months is the earliest FDA-approved age of implantation. In actuality, many children are being implanted even at six months of age. The earlier the age of implantation, the better the results.

In some ways, being born hearing-impaired and then receiving a cochlear implant is like being born premature. For the first two years of a prematurely born child's life, doctors frequently age-adjust developmental milestones based on the day the child should have been born, rather than the day the child was born. So a nine-month-old who was born three months early is six months old age-adjusted, and has the three months of prematurity to catch up. The day the cochlear implant is activated is the day the hearing system is born. If that day is when the child is six months old, then he or she has to catch up six months, plus the five months of auditory development time that was lost in the womb. If a child gets a cochlear implant at two years of age, he or she has twenty-nine months of hearing to catch up on. Obviously, if your child is deaf, you don't want to give his or her peers and future competitors at school, jobs, etc., that much of a head start!

If no sound has gone through the hearing system during the first five years of life, the brain's auditory pathways will be either absent or very poorly developed. If a cochlear implant is placed in a patient after the time for these pathways to develop has passed, it will not provide much function at all. The best we expect is for the patient to have some awareness of sound, but little or no ability to understand speech. Some patients in this category still elect to have a cochlear implant placed, hoping this will improve their speech reading skills, but these patients will never be able to understand spoken language without additional cues coming through visual input and speech reading.

The Process of Receiving a Cochlear Implant

A multistep, multidisciplinary approach is used to determine who is a good candidate to receive a cochlear implant. This involves many of the team members discussed in the section on care providers. At a high level, the process of receiving an implant includes:

- Assessment
- Surgery
- After-surgery medical care
- Audiological follow-up
- Additional therapy (speech/language/auditory-verbal therapy)
- Educational adjustments

FDA Criteria for Cochlear Implantation

FDA guidelines for cochlear implantation for children are as follows:

- Aged twelve months to eighteen years

- Must have profound sensorineural hearing impairment in both ears (speech reception threshold/pure tone average rated at "not useful," i.e. 90 decibels hearing level (HL) or worse)

- Limited benefit from appropriate binaural hearing aids

- Children older than five years must score 30 percent or less on sentence recognition tests under best-aided conditions (best-fit hearing aids in place)

- High motivation and appropriate expectations from family

FDA guidelines for cochlear implantation for adults are:

- Must have moderate to profound sensorineural hearing impairment in both ears; speech reception threshold/pure tone average rated greater than 70 dB HL or scoring less than 60 percent on sentence recognition tests under best-aided conditions (best-fit hearing aids in place), or 40 to 60 percent if they are enrolled in a clinical trial

- A desire to be a part of the hearing world

In addition, the following guidelines apply to all candidates:

- No medical contraindications may be present (e.g., no cochlear aplasia, no active middle ear infection, eighth cranial nerve must be present).

- Communication between patients, families, schools, audiologists, therapists, and surgeons is required.

Cochlear Implant Candidacy Assessment

The procedures involved in assessing an individual patient for cochlear implantation differ from clinic to clinic. Larger clinics are integrated; that is, they can provide all of the necessary assessments using providers at their clinic. Other, smaller clinics may refer patients to outside providers for portions of the assessments.

Cochlear Implant Medical Appointment

All cochlear implant candidates must be seen for an initial candidacy evaluation by the implant surgeon. This appointment will focus on current and past hearing status and overall health history. The surgeon will also inquire about the cochlear implant candidate's vaccination status. It is essential that all cochlear implant candidates have up-to-date meningitis vaccinations. Individuals who are cochlear implant candidates have a higher rate of meningitis, a life-threatening bacterial infection, than the general population, regardless of whether they actually receive a cochlear implant.

In addition to this history, the cochlear implant surgeon will require a CT scan to assess the inner ear. The CT scan will confirm the path of the facial nerve, confirm the presence of the auditory nerve, and identify any cochlear malformations or ossification (bony growth within the cochlea) that may make implantation difficult. Children under the age of three and others who are incapable of keeping still during the period of the exam may require sedation for the CT to take place.

Cochlear Implant Candidacy Audiological Evaluation

Audiologic unaided and aided testing will be performed to assess hearing ability and to determine hearing aid benefit. In infants, this generally includes a behavioral assessment as well as sedated auditory brainstem response/auditory steady-state response testing. In addition to obtaining unaided and aided hearing thresholds, adults are assessed for word recognition ability with the use of power hearing aids. Topics that the audiologist will review with the cochlear implant candidate or the candidate's parents generally include:

- An overall review of how cochlear implants work and how they differ from hearing aids
- Expectations for performance with device use
- Choice of implant devices for use and how they function
- Cochlear implant programming follow-up and schedule of appointments
- Educational placement
- Rehabilitative service
- Other evaluations needed to complete candidacy work-up
- Maintenance of cochlear implant equipment

Cochlear Implant Candidacy Speech Assessment

It is important to establish a baseline evaluation of the patient's speech and language development prior to receiving the implant surgery. Some patients who receive cochlear implants may have other issues above and beyond their hearing impairment that may adversely affect their speech development, such as a cleft palate, oral-motor issues, or apraxia. In addition, having a full speech assessment done in children prior to surgery will result in a report that the parents can use to get appropriate audiology and language support services from their school district, either through an early-intervention Individualized Family Service Plan (IFSP) if the child is three or under, or an Individualized Education Program (IEP) if the child is over the age of three.

Other Potential Cochlear Implant Candidacy Assessments

Other assessments included by some cochlear implant centers include psychological evaluation, physical therapy/occupational therapy evaluation, and vision assessment.

Cochlear Implant Surgery

Cochlear implant surgery is always performed under general anesthesia. The patient is placed on his or her back, with the head turned so that the ear receiving the implant is facing up. A small amount of hair is shaved, and an outline is traced around the receiver/stimulator area on the side of the head where the implant will be placed. The placement of the receiver/stimulator needs to be far enough away from the ear that it won't interfere with the behind-the-ear speech processor, but not so far away that it is likely to come off every time a child is placed into a car seat.

An incision is created behind the ear, which allows the surgeon access to the layers of tissue between the skin and the bone where the cochlear implant receiver/stimulator will be placed. An incision is cut through skin and muscle to expose the bone with its periosteum, a tough protective covering.

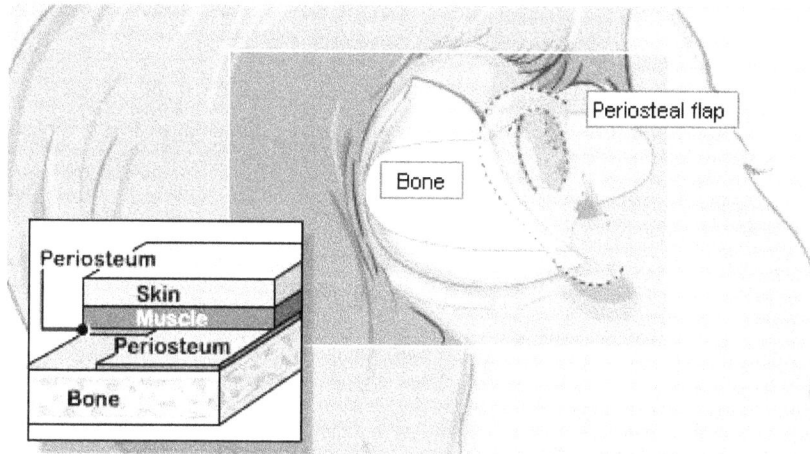

Next, a flap is cut into the periosteum. Pockets are created between the periosteal layer and the bone. These pockets are where the cochlear implant receiver/stimulator and electrode will be placed.

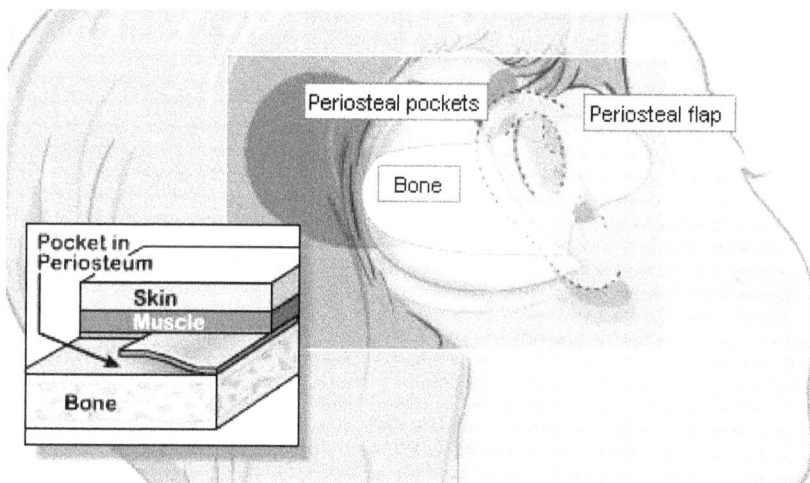

The surgeon then creates a shallow well in the bone to ensure that there is enough room for the cochlear implant receiver/stimulator to be well-seated. To drill the well, the surgeon uses a small device similar to a dental drill. A template is used to guide the well drilling. After the well is made, the surgeon then creates tie-down holes that help secure the implant in its correct position.

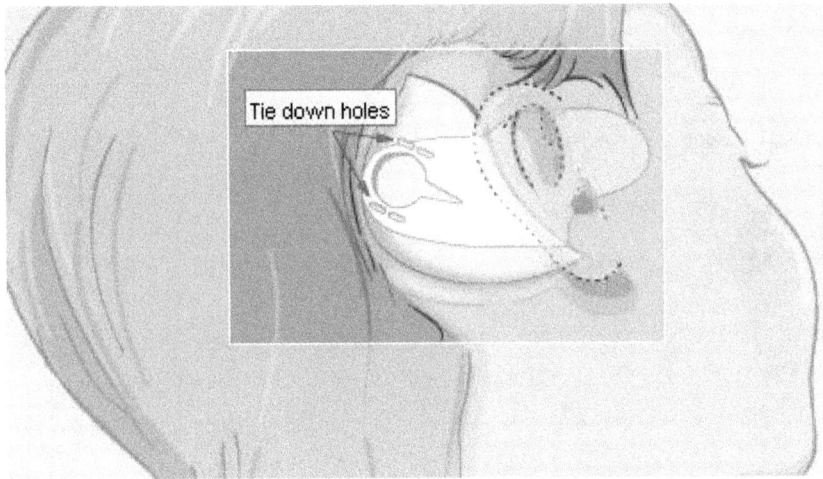

Once the well and tie-down holes have been drilled into the mastoid, the surgeon performs a mastoidectomy, removing bone from the mastoid space behind the ear canal. Next, the surgeon creates a facial recess, which is any tiny channel that gives the surgeon access to the patient's middle ear and a visual perspective of the facial nerve. Then a small hole, called a cochleostomy, is drilled through the fragile wall of the cochlea. The cochleostomy is the hole that allows the electrode array of the cochlear implant electrode to be threaded.

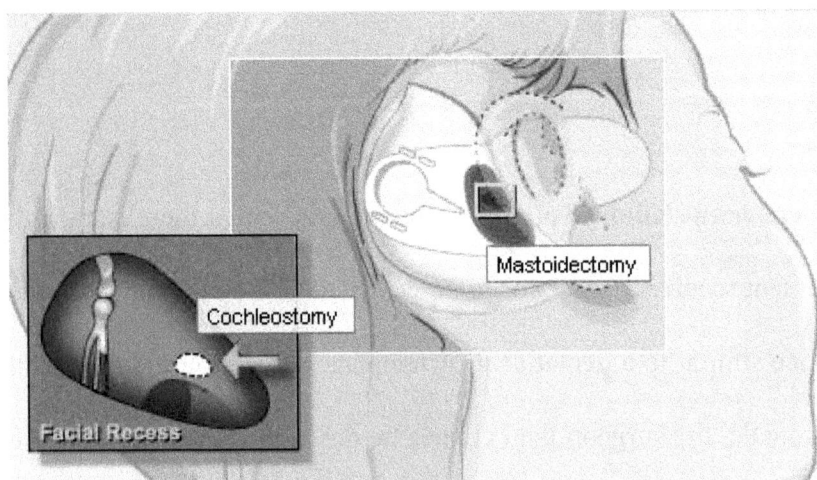

The electrode array is held in a semi-straight position with a stylet and guided through the cochleostomy. Once the electrode array is inside the cochlea, the stylet is removed and the electrode array curls into the inner wall of the cochlea. The implant receiver/stimulator is placed in the previously created pocket in the mastoid and is secured with sutures through the tie-down holes. The device is tested electronically in the operating room before the patient wakes up to ensure it is intact and capable of stimulating the auditory nerve.

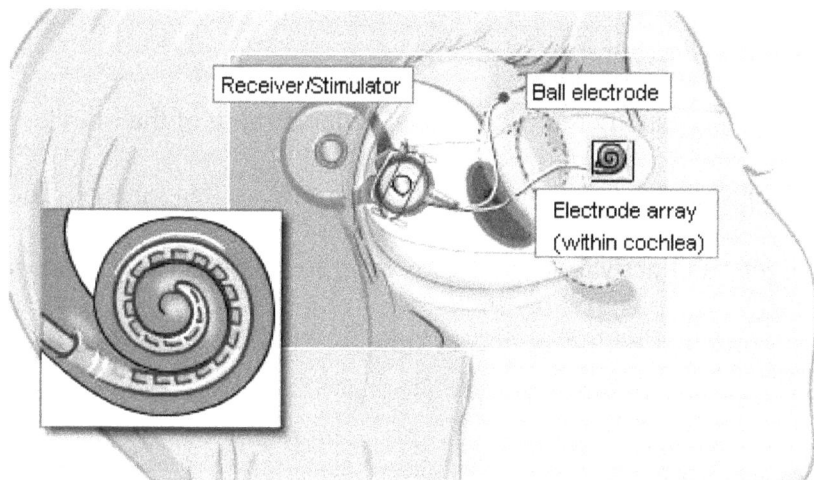

The incision is closed and the head is bandaged overnight. Generally, cochlear implant surgery does not require an overnight hospital stay. In most cases, the bandages are removed the following morning, and the sutures are removed ten days after surgery.

For an animated description of cochlear implant surgery, please go to http://www.letthemhear.org/hearing/implants.php# and click on "View the animations to learn about implant surgery."

Cochlear Implant Post-Surgery Medical Care

Medical care after cochlear implant surgery is generally fairly minimal. Unless the patient is under the age of one year or has some known concurrent medical issue, such as a heart condition, it is most likely that this surgery will be performed at an ambulatory surgery center and the patient will be sent home as soon as an hour or so after waking up from the general anesthesia. Pain medication such as Tylenol with codeine may be prescribed, but many people don't feel the need to take it. Occasionally, tinnitus or balance problems may occur or worsen immediately after the surgery, but these symptoms usually subside fairly quickly. Children typically bounce back within a day or two. One or two post-operative appointments will be required to check the incision sites and ensure that there is no infection.

Cochlear Implant Audiological Follow-up

Cochlear implant recipients usually return for initial programming of their devices (known as initial activation or stimulation) about three to four weeks after surgery. The waiting period between surgery and activation used to be five to six weeks, but studies have shown that there is no problem with a period of time as short as a few days to a week.

At the activation appointment, the audiologist will fit the external equipment to make sure that all components are appropriate and functioning. Activation appointments are frequently done over two days for a single device, or four days for simultaneous bilateral implantation. This is because there is a fatigue factor when the brain receives all of this auditory input for the first time, or after an absence of auditory input for postlingually deafened individuals. In addition, there is quite a bit of new information to cover, such as care and use of the devices and accessories, and it can be overwhelming to review all of this in one day.

The initial activation begins by connecting the cochlear implant speech processor to a computer for programming. An impedance measurement of the electrodes is completed to confirm that all electrodes are functioning. Initially, the responses from the auditory nerve that were obtained in the operating room following surgery are used to help define the first settings. These responses are called neural response telemetry (NRT) or imaging (NRI).

Next, the audiologist, with the help of the cochlear implant recipient, determines what values constitute the softest sound (T level) and a comfortably loud sound (C or M level) for specific contact points (called electrodes) for the cochlear implant. These values will be used to create the first program, or "map".

With young children, this can be a difficult task. Often the NRT responses are used to create the shape of the map, and the speech processor is turned on at a very soft level and gradually increased until the child shows some reaction to the sound stimulation. Eye widening, quieting, smiling, or even crying are typical reactions that are seen in response to the sound. It is important to remember that a congenitally hearing-impaired child has never heard before, and the experience can be frightening at first. The main goal at the initial activation of a young child's cochlear implant is to get a comfortable level of sound in, ensuring that the child will wear the device consistently and comfortably. Overstimulating the child at the initial activation can result in the child rejecting the device.

Once the first map has been created, three progressively louder maps are created for the individual to work through until the next programming session. The auditory nerve and brain can only take so much stimulation at first, but adaptation to the sound occurs quickly, and the individual will require more and more power. Once the initial cochlear implant activation programming has been completed and the programs have been downloaded to the processor, the external equipment function is reviewed with the recipient.

Over a patient's lifetime, the cochlear implant will require different programs to function optimally. Ongoing follow-up audiology visits will be necessary to update the maps, assist the recipient with specific needs that he or she may have related to the cochlear implant, and evaluate performance with the device.

Additionally, the cochlear implant audiologist will help in determining whether the implant recipient is an appropriate candidate for aural rehabilitation and/or speech and language therapy. New implant users, both children and adults, often find that one-on-one therapy initiated shortly after the cochlear implant is activated is extremely beneficial to their device learning curve. The therapist can assist in establishing realistic goals and expectations, help the individual to maximize his or her listening potential, assist with IEP goal definition, and provide home program exercises. Even families of children who are already receiving therapy services at school find that adjunct services in the private sector are quite beneficial. This is especially true when the services are provided by an integrated cochlear implant center, which allows for excellent communication and continuity of care between all of the implant team members.

Cochlear Implant Therapy

Several types of therapeutic services are available to help children with cochlear implants acquire age-appropriate speech, language, developmental, and social skills. According to the Children's Hearing Institute:

> Children implanted early, who do not have other significant developmental disabilities, and when coupled with intensive post-implantation speech language therapy, may acquire age appropriate speech, language, developmental and social skills.

It is important to begin therapy immediately following initial activation of the device, because your child will be hearing many new sounds that he or she has never heard before. Speech/language therapy is necessary to help your child identify and understand the new sounds he or she is hearing, and to naturally combine the various components of communication, including listening, speech, language, reading, and thinking. Many cochlear implant clinics believe speech therapy is so important that they require parents of young children to sign an agreement laying out the plan for rehabilitation following surgery. You, as the parent and the coach, will play an integral role in the habilitation of your child's speech and language skills. Often you will be involved in the therapy sessions in order to become educated and trained on how to enable continued learning in the home.

Auditory-verbal therapy (AVT) is one therapy option for children with hearing loss. It emphasizes the use of spoken language through early identification of hearing loss, early and appropriate amplification, and intensive speech and language therapy, in which the parent serves as the primary language model for the child. The child is taught to use the hearing he or she has to understand speech and learn to talk. The goal of AVT is for hearing-impaired children to grow up in a regular learning environment, which will allow them to become independent, participating, and contributing adults in mainstream society. AVT is a parent-centered approach, and parents are taught how to interact with their children. AVT follows a strict set of guidelines, emphasizing natural conversation and the use of spoken language. The parent, therapist, and child engage in play activities that teach the child to use his or her amplified residual hearing to learn auditory-verbal communication like children with normal hearing.

Other Assistive Technology

Anyone who wears a hearing device knows that one significant disadvantage is that sometimes, unwanted sounds are amplified in addition to speech. For a hearing-impaired child in a classroom or an adult in the workplace, this can prove to be a major handicap in locations where they spend a lot of time.

Classrooms typically have very bad acoustics. Sounds from echoes, scraping chairs, and background chatter can make it difficult for a hearing-impaired child to understand the teacher. Even if the student is seated near the front of the classroom and the teacher is catering to his or her needs (directly facing the child and speaking clearly), the child can still miss a lot. The audiological term for this issue is "signal-to-noise ratio," frequently abbreviated as S/N. The closer the decibel level of the signal to the noise, the more of a problem it is for the hearing-impaired individual to understand the signal (i.e. the speech) over the background noise. Classroom acoustics generally have signal-to-noise ratios of +7 decibels or worse.

Workplaces can be even worse than classrooms. Very few people work in offices by themselves, with doors they can close anytime they want. Far more frequent work locations are warehouses, retail environments, restaurants, or "cubicle farms." People talking, phones ringing, file drawers opening and closing, and cash registers can all create unwanted background noise that hinders hearing-impaired working adults from getting their jobs done. Even in optimal work environments, group meetings with multiple people talking simultaneously make understanding who is speaking and what they are saying a very difficult task. Hearing-impaired individuals are entitled to reasonable accommodations under the Americans with Disabilities Act (ADA) in order to lessen the effect that their hearing impairment has on their job function.

Fortunately, a number of assistive listening device (ALD) systems are available to help hearing-impaired students and employees. The four major ALD systems are the FM system, the sound-field system, the Loop system, and CART. Most of these systems are relatively inexpensive, and therefore would be considered a reasonable accommodation under the ADA.

FM Systems

The FM system uses a wireless transmitter to broadcast a signal throughout a given area. The size of the broadcast area is determined by the power of the transmitter, with an auditorium typically being the maximum practical size.

The main speaker wears the FM microphone and transmitter, and the hearing-impaired individual wears an FM receiver. The receiver is typically extremely small. If the hearing-impaired individual wears a hearing device, the FM receiver typically is connected directly to the bottom of the hearing aid. The portion that connects with the device is generally referred to as a "boot." FM systems may also be directly attached to many newer cochlear implant or Baha devices through a mechanism referred to as DAI, for "direct auditory input." If the hearing-impaired individual doesn't wear hearing aids, headphones may be used.

The batteries in the speaker's transmitter are typically rechargeable, and the entire unit can be placed in a base station every night for recharging. The latest development in FM system technology uses the Bluetooth standard to allow cell phone communications, for example, to be routed through the FM system directly to the hearing aid, rather than having the phone up to the ear. If the FM system is being used in a classroom with more than one hearing-impaired student, each student's receiver can be set to pick up a single microphone transmission device.

FM system operation is extremely simple. Both the speaker and the hearing-impaired individual turn on their respective components. The speaker speaks into a small microphone. The microphone is often worn on the lapel, about five to seven inches from the speaker's mouth. The microphone is very sensitive and can pick up sounds like fabric or jewelry rubbing against it. The speaker's voice is then carried without any distortion to the hearing-impaired individual's hearing device or headphones. In the case of a hearing device, the sound is then processed using the programs in the hearing-impaired individual's hearing aid that are specifically tailored to their hearing impairment. For example, if a hearing-impaired individual has worse hearing in the upper frequencies, the hearing aids will take the FM signal from a high-frequency female's voice and amplify that more loudly than a lower-frequency male's voice.

Using the FM system, the hearing-impaired individual can hear the speaker clearly anywhere in the broadcast area. The range of the system is ten to ninety feet, depending on the limitations of the particular technology selected. Therefore, it is possible for the speaker to physically leave the room and the hearing-impaired individual to still be able to hear what the speaker is saying. If the speaker has his or her back to the hearing-impaired individual, while writing on a chalkboard for example, his or her voice will still be clearly heard by the student wearing the FM receiver.

One significant advantage of an FM system is its portability. The transmitter is small and can be used in any room. No permanent installation is required, and the hearing-impaired individual has his or her own receiving device that easily goes with him or her from speaker to speaker and room to room. In the case of FM system use by a student, given that most single-teacher education ends by fifth grade, this feature is especially important for middle school and high school students. It is also important for university students, who are likely to hear lectures more clearly in large amphitheaters with poor acoustics and large quantities of background noise.

The FM system can be used to amplify the human voice, a movie soundtrack, or another audio source, making it ideal for classroom use. In kindergarten classrooms, teachers frequently remove the microphone and pass it from child to child during activities such as group reading and circle time. This also works in group meeting settings, where the microphone can be passed from speaker to speaker to assist the hearing-impaired employee in following the group conversation.

In the United States, if an FM system or any other piece of assistive technology is required in order for a student to receive a Free Appropriate Public Education (FAPE), then the school district is obligated to purchase the FM system under the Individuals with Disabilities Education Act (IDEA). Some children with hearing impairments have FM system usage written into a 504 plan; other children, who require more substantial modifications to their education environments as a result of their hearing impairments, have FM system usage listed as one component of their specialized education requirements in an IEP.

Sound-Field Systems

Sound-field systems are similar to FM systems, in that they both use FM radio waves to transmit the desired sound. Sound-field systems come in two varieties: a personal sound-field system, which uses an amplifier that sits on a child's desk, similar to a boom box; or a classroom sound-field system, in which several small, wall-mounted amplifiers are used to amplify sound all over the classroom.

A personal sound-field system is intended for the use of the hearing-impaired user only. It is generally portable and configured in a boom box-type package that can be carried from classroom to classroom. Whereas FM systems and personal sound-field systems only benefit those students possessing the receivers, classroom sound-field systems are designed to overcome poor classroom acoustics through multiple, small wall-mounted amplifiers, thereby benefiting all of the students in the classroom.

With a classroom sound-field system, the teacher wears a small microphone, and his or her voice is broadcast to loudspeakers placed strategically throughout the classroom. The sound of the teacher's voice is amplified enough to compensate for background noise. Students in the back of the room can hear as clearly as those in the front. These systems are less portable than the FM systems due to the physical installation of the loudspeakers, which are generally anchored into the classroom walls. These systems are generally only used for children in elementary school, as it is unusual for children past sixth grade to receive all of their class instruction in a single room.

Sound-field systems are useful for students with mild to moderate hearing impairment. They also provide benefits to the teacher. Teachers can maintain voice contact with every student in the classroom without raising their voices. All students in the classroom are better able to concentrate on what the teacher is saying. It has been demonstrated that children with ADHD, without any hearing impairment, benefit from the installation of classroom sound-field systems because they are better able to focus on the teacher's verbal instructions.

Although it is possible to use a sound-field system in a workplace setting, because it requires physical installation of speakers, it restricts the rooms in which the hearing-impaired employee can use this technology, which limits its benefit.

Loop System

Loop systems have been used for many years, but are generally more popular in Europe than in America. Based on telephone technology, they are time-proven systems for assisting individuals with hearing impairment in picking up speech in areas known to be noisy.

Loop systems use a cable that circles (or "loops") the listening area. The loop can be any size, and can be placed anywhere. It could be around a classroom, an auditorium, a table for conference work, or even a car. The speaker speaks into a microphone, and the signal is amplified and fed through the loop. Listeners receive the signal through specially equipped hearing aids that receive electromagnetic signals. These hearing aids are very common and have a built-in telecoil switch, known as a "T switch."

Most current hearing aid technology and cochlear implant technology utilizes integrated telecoils. For people with such technology, this system is very easy to use. There is no need for a separate receiver, as with FM systems. The user must only switch his or her device into the telecoil program.

Loop systems are relatively easy to install and therefore economical. Several small looped systems could easily be installed in various school areas, such as the library check-out desk, the office, and anywhere that the hearing-impaired student needs to communicate effectively.

CART

For students or employees with severe hearing impairments, the Communication Access Realtime Translation (CART) system can be of great benefit to the classroom lecture or group meeting environment. Originally used for court transcription, CART has found new applications as an educational tool.

A specially trained CART operator uses a transcription machine to record all spoken text. The text is either displayed on a computer monitor or projected on a screen. If broadband Internet access is available, the CART operator does not have to be in the same room, or even on the same continent. If the spoken text is transmitted in real time over the Internet, the CART operator can be overseas. The ability to use lower-cost overseas CART operators has increased the popularity of its use in the United States.

One benefit of the CART system is that all speech is recorded, not just that of the main speaker. In the classroom setting, this allows the hearing-impaired student to keep up with comments from other students and participate more fully in group classroom conversations. In a group meeting setting, this allows the hearing-impaired employee to follow a question-and-answer session following a main speaker's presentation.

Another benefit inherent to CART is that there is a written record of everything said in the classroom or at the conference. These written transcripts can later be used and reviewed as either study or training aids.

In the school system, CART systems are usually only used in high school and college or university-level institutions. They are also frequently used at conferences involving an audience that may contain hearing-impaired individuals. The cost is greater than that of other systems because of the need to pay the transcriptionist. Hearing-impaired individuals who have had access to CART, however, often prefer it to other assistive listening devices, because CART allows them to more easily and visually follow what is going on in conversations in the classroom and other group environments, which in turn allows them to play a more active role.

Service Animals

Everybody is familiar with seeing-eye dogs, those wonderful, dedicated animals that allow the blind to lead independent lives. Less well-known are the dogs and other animals trained to help people with other disabilities. These animals, generally referred to as "service animals," help open up opportunities to thousands of disabled people.

Service animals can offer assistance both inside and outside the home. They can help people with physical impairments in such tasks as opening and closing doors, pulling a wheelchair, and getting objects that are out of reach. They can also provide balance and guidance to people who have difficulty walking. There are also animals trained for special purposes such as classroom assistance. These dogs can help teachers or therapists working with physically or emotionally handicapped children. The dog provides motivation to the children and can be a calming influence in the classroom.

Of most interest to the hearing-impaired community are dogs that are specially trained to assist people with hearing impairments. Hearing dogs receive instruction that teaches them to respond to common household sounds like the doorbell, the telephone, a smoke alarm, or a knock at the door. When the dog hears one of these sounds, or any others it has been trained for, it responds by alerting its hearing-impaired master, who can ask the dog to show him or her where the sound is coming from.

Hearing dog training dates back to 1974. Agnes McGrath, a dog trainer in Minnesota, was asked by a hearing-impaired woman to train a dog for her. The hearing-impaired woman had previously had a dog that was informally trained to react to sound, but that dog had died of old age.

Ms. McGrath agreed to do it, and received funding from the local Lions Clubs chapter to train six dogs. Afterward, the project was taken over by the American Humane Association. It received a grant for a four-year pilot project conducted in Colorado. As a result of that project, the International Hearing Dog organization was formed.

On the East Coast, a similar organization called National Education for Assistance Dog

Services (NEADS) has been operating since 1976. NEADS trains service dogs for all purposes except sight. There are many other hearing dog organizations throughout the world.

Hearing dogs are typically reserved for people with severe to profound hearing impairment. For these people, a hearing dog can make a significant improvement in their ability to live independently. Not only does the dog improve their safety by alerting them to dangerous sounds they cannot hear, the dog gives them increased mobility and independence. There are also emotional advantages to having a hearing dog.

Hearing dogs are initially trained to respond to all the usual obedience commands, such as "sit" and "come." If the dog is to be assigned to a person who uses sign language, the dog will be trained to respond to sign language in addition to voice commands. Dogs can also receive additional specialized training to help hearing-impaired individuals who have additional disabilities.

Hearing dogs are usually selected from animal shelters. Trainers are looking for friendly, intelligent young dogs or pups. These otherwise unwanted dogs are given the opportunity to lead happy, productive lives by becoming hearing dogs. Hearing dogs can be any size, but are most often small or medium, because they are frequently trained to nudge or jump on hearing-impaired individuals to alert them to sounds, and getting repeatedly nudged by a Saint Bernard or Great Dane might be a bit overwhelming for some people. Also, breeds such as Dalmatians and Poodles (which are prone to genetic hearing defects) or herding/hunting animals are generally avoided, as they typically do not have the appropriate innate dispositions to make good hearing dogs.

After the initial selection, the dog has a medical examination to make sure it is in good health, and is generally spayed or neutered. Once the dog has received a clean bill of health, it proceeds to initial obedience training, followed by training specific to the person it is being placed with. Training can last anywhere from four to eight months. Aside from basic obedience skills, the dog has to be socially trained not to be aggressive, not to beg, and to avoid unnecessary barking and jumping on people.

After basic skills are mastered, hearing dogs are trained to respond to up to twenty common sounds, such as the phone ringing or a knock on the door. When the hearing dog hears a sound it has been trained to respond to, it will alert its master to the sound, then lead him or her to the source of the sound. For sounds that the dog has been trained indicate danger, the dog reacts a little bit differently. Again it will get the attention of its master, but this time it will drop to the floor to indicate that it is dangerous to go toward the source of the sound.

After obedience training and sound training, the dog has to go through a final stage of training in the recipient's home. This part of the training can take about three months. The trainer supervises the dog's adjustment to its new home and teaches the recipient how to care for his or her dog.

On successful completion of the training program, the dog can wear a special orange vest and collar identifying its status as a working service dog. If registered with a service dog organization, the dog may also have an ID card, which shows its picture and briefly explains the special rights it has as a service animal. These rights include access to public facilities such as restaurants, shopping centers, and movie theaters.

Key Takeaways

1. Hearing devices have come a long way during the last 50 years. They are now fully digital and can be customized to the person's specific hearing needs.

2. If hearing aids are recommended for your child, establishing a hearing aid routine

right from the beginning will aid in your child's acceptance of the devices. Remember, you are the boss of your child's hearing aids!

3. The goal of hearing aid use is that your child will wear the aids the majority of his or her waking hours; you may have to work up to this in smaller increments of time.

4. Children pull their hearing aids out, or they fall out, for a number of reasons. There are simple ways to help keep the hearing aids in, such as using wig tape, "huggies," or caps. Inevitably, though, the hearing aids will fall out, so it is extremely important to have a safeguard in place, such as fishing line or critter clips that help to keep the hearing aids from getting lost.

5. Children with single-sided deafness or unilateral hearing loss have difficulty in a number of areas and should be aided. Hearing with two ears is always better than hearing with one.

6. A bone-anchored prosthetic device is a surgically implanted hearing device that is appropriate for individuals with conductive hearing impairment, unilateral or bilateral; profound sensorineural hearing impairment in one ear and normal hearing in the other; or mixed hearing impairment.

7. A cochlear implant is a surgically implanted device that sends electrical stimulation directly to the auditory nerve and can bring hearing to profoundly hearing-impaired individuals.

8. Determining who is a good cochlear implant candidate is a multidisciplinary process and involves a number of professionals and evaluations. Strict criteria must be met for an individual to be considered a cochlear implant candidate.

9. Once an individual receives a cochlear implant, ongoing audiological follow-up and rehabilitation are imperative to a successful outcome.

10. Other assistive technology can be used in conjunction with hearing devices and can allow for better speech understanding, such as FM systems, sound-field systems, loop systems, and CART.

Chapter 6

Treatment Funding Options

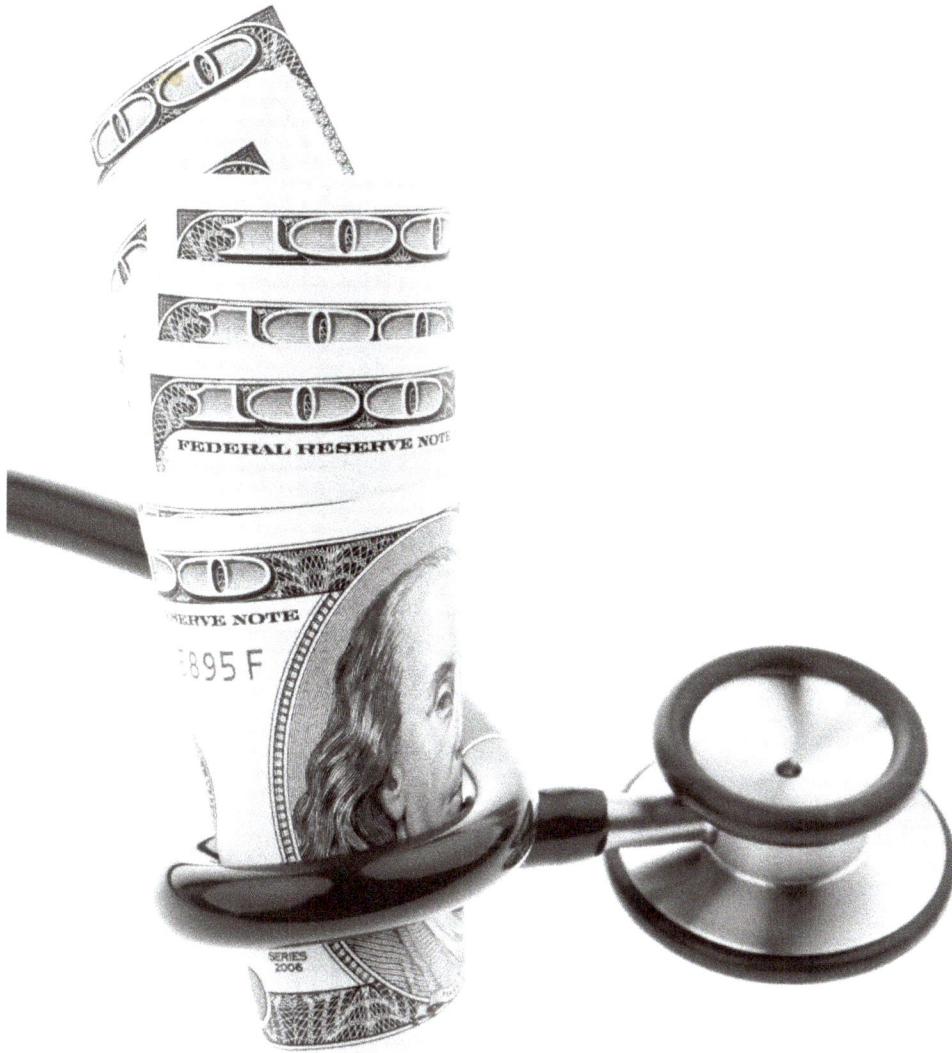

Introduction

Treatment for hearing impairment-related issues and assistive listening devices can be extremely expensive. Some examples of prices, in U.S. dollars:

- Digital hearing aids: $2,900 for one, or $5,800 for two

- Baha implantation: $14,000 to $18,000 for one ear

- Cochlear implant: $38,000 to $60,000 for one; $68,000 to over $100,000 for two

- FM system: $600 to $2,100

- Speech therapy: $95 per hour and up

Because most families cannot afford to simply write a check and pay for these items out of their own funds, it is extremely important to understand the funding options that are available in order to obtain the equipment and services that your medical service providers recommend.

Types of Health Insurance

Many different types of health insurance are available. It is extremely important to understand what insurance options may be available to you and what restrictions may apply to that insurance with respect to preexisting conditions.

Group Health Insurance

More than 200 million Americans have access to group health insurance benefits. When it comes to health insurance, employer-based or group coverage is almost always the best option. Group insurance is most commonly obtained either directly through a job, or as the dependent of someone who has obtained the group health insurance through a job.

Another source of group health insurance is association coverage, which is sponsored by established large groups of individuals such as unions or the AARP. There have been some fraudulent schemes involving association coverage, but many reputable association coverage options are available. Carefully investigate the credentials of any association whose policy you are considering purchasing; this should include checking with the Better Business Bureau.

When you have group health insurance, either through a job or an association, there is no direct contract between you and the insurer. There are two contracts: one between the group and the insurer, and a second between you and the group. Group health insurance coverage for issues relating to hearing impairment can range from extremely good to nonexistent, depending on the plan. It is important to read the summary plan bulletin document, which will tell you what items are covered or not covered for your plan. Recently, UnitedHealthcare, a large and diversified health company, announced that it would add coverage for hearing aids to many plans as part of the expansion of the Americans with Disabilities Act of 2009.[7]

The best feature of group insurance is that the insurer cannot permanently refuse to provide coverage due to the hearing impairment being a preexisting condition. If you have been uninsured for more than sixty-three days at the time you start on a new group plan, there may be a waiting period of up to eighteen months before you will receive coverage for any medical condition you have prior to your insurance start date. However, you will be fully covered to the

---

[7]

http://www.uhc.com/news_room/health_care_reform/americans_with_disabilities_act_(ada)_protections_e
xpanded_for_2009/relatedinformation/7ff2b6c25a355210VgnVCM2000003010b10a____.htm

extent of the plan limits when the specified waiting period is over.

Group insurance is also available to individuals who are self-employed, as well as their dependents, depending on the rules of the group. It is possible to get insurance for a group of one. About a dozen states allow the self-employed to buy into the small group market, which affords more protections and cheaper rates. If you are self-employed, there are tax advantages to obtaining insurance through this market. Individual insurance purchases by the same individual do not receive preferential tax treatment. It is also possible to get group insurance through human resources outsourcing agencies such as Insperity or Gevity HR, which include handling all benefits as part of their contractual relationships with businesses.

Individual Health Insurance

With individual health insurance, you have a direct contract with an insurer for insurance just for you, or for you and your dependents. Unlike group health insurance, in which everyone in a group is covered regardless of their health status, individual health insurance is affected by the concept known as "adverse selection," which means that individuals who know or suspect that they have health issues are more likely to seek out individual insurance when group insurance is not available. Thus, the pool of people being insured with individual plans, in contrast to group plans, includes more people with a high need for costly health care. As a result of adverse selection, individual health insurance policies frequently cover substantially less than group health plans, and your health insurance dollar will buy you less coverage in the individual health insurance plan market.

Individual health insurance plan premiums vary widely depending on the state, the person's age, and the specific benefits. The average premium for family coverage on a comprehensive plan can easily exceed $10,000 per year. There is a wide range of products in the individual market, from catastrophic-only coverage to comprehensive health plans, as well as products that cover only a specific disease, like cancer. The most important thing to remember is to look carefully at what each policy covers, and under what circumstances that coverage is available.

The main difference between individual insurance and group insurance is that except under very specific circumstances, individual insurers are allowed to refuse to accept your application for coverage. If they do accept an application, they are allowed to temporarily or permanently exclude benefits related to conditions that they do not wish to provide coverage for. Typically, exclusions for an existing hearing impairment under individual health insurance policies are permanent. In the alternative, some insurers may offer to cover the condition, but boost the price of the policy premium. As of September 23, 2010, children cannot be excluded from any insurance plans, including individual plans, due to preexisting conditions.

Medical debt causes a big share of bankruptcies, even for people who have insurance. The problem in those cases is mostly due to a lack of insurance protection when a serious health condition strikes. When shopping for individual health insurance, low premiums may be attractive at first, but what really matters is your total cost of health care under the plan. The total cost includes a combination of your premiums plus your likely out-of-pocket spending on health care below the deductible, plus all copays and any costs for care that is either explicitly excluded or has a limited amount of coverage, if you will exceed the limit. While it may be tempting, don't shop for individual health insurance based on premium alone.

When you are shopping for individual health insurance, where you live is important for several reasons. The first is that each state has different laws regarding your rights to purchase insurance. Buying coverage in the individual market is easier in some states, such as Maine, Massachusetts, New Jersey, New York, and Vermont, because those states have passed laws protecting residents and requiring insurers to provide them with the opportunity to purchase health insurance, regardless of their health condition.

Other factors to investigate include whether or not the policy is guaranteed renewable, which means you have the right to renew the policy annually. If a policy is not guaranteed renewable, your policy could be cancelled at the end of the policy period if you get sick or get in an accident. Another factor is how the insurer calculates premium increases. For the past decade, the rise in the cost of medical care and health insurance premiums has far exceeded the rate of inflation. In recent years, some plans in some states have attempted to raise premiums by up to almost 40 percent per year. When you are shopping for an individual health insurance plan, it is important to ask what procedure the company uses to calculate yearly premium increases.

If individual health insurance is your only option, it is important to understand the rules of your specific policy, including what is covered and when. Individual policies generally don't offer the robust coverage found in group policies. Talk to an insurance broker, and ask the following questions:

- *What does the policy cover?* Individual health insurance plans often contain blanket exclusions eliminating benefits for many conditions, including hearing impairment.

- *Are there policy coverage limits?* Lifetime limits are currently not an issue but could be put back in to place by a change in legislation.

- *Is there a catastrophic cap?* Many insurance plans have "catastrophic caps," which place a limit on your total financial obligation in a given year. For example, a policy might have a catastrophic cap of $4,000 per individual and $8,000 per family. Many plans have different caps for in-network services versus services that are received out of network. Depending on the policy, you may have a higher or lower out-of-pocket individual or family maximum.

- *Can I add a spouse if I get married or a child if I give birth or adopt?* Some individual plans require you to reapply for coverage, including a new analysis of your own medical status, if you wish to add members to your individual health insurance plan. Ask if there are circumstances under which you would need to reapply for coverage.

- *What does the insurance company say about annual or any other rate increases?* On what basis will the company raise the monthly premium you pay? Healthcare reform and state insurance commissioners have done very little to regulate health insurance rate increases, and some individuals have seen regular double-digit rate increases as the economy has worsened and healthy people have dropped individual plans, increasing the self-selection of high-risk people in the insurance pool.

COBRA Insurance

When you leave a job, whether by voluntarily quitting or being laid off, you may be able to extend health insurance benefits you received from the job via a federal law called COBRA. This law allows you to continue in your employer's group plan for eighteen months (in some cases longer), and it may be a good option during transitions between group health insurance plans, or while you search for the right individual insurance policy. You'll have to pay the full cost of the health insurance plan, which may have been previously subsidized by your employer, plus a 2 percent administrative fee. Some people are astonished to find that the cost of this insurance for a family may exceed $1,000 per month.

Government Health Insurance

In most states, some form of insurance from the government is available. However, this government health insurance is nothing like the universal coverage that is available in Canada and Europe. Frequently, eligibility for a government health insurance plan depends on very strict guidelines, including your income, your assets, and whether you are disabled. Furthermore, having a government health insurance plan as your only source of insurance all but restricts you to universities or other extremely large health centers for treatment. This is because the amount of reimbursement by the government under these health insurance plans is so low (frequently 20 cents on the dollar or less) that only large universities and nonprofits with endowments have the financial means to absorb the significant losses that treating these patients creates. These large centers frequently have correspondingly long waiting lists.

All states have government-funded Medicaid programs available for children, usually defined as individuals under the age of twenty-one. These programs are partially financed by the federal government, but are instituted on a state-by-state basis. In order to receive federal funding for their state Medicaid programs, all states are mandated to offer at least a unilateral cochlear implant to individuals under the age of twenty-one. Cochlear implants are not mandated for adults on Medicaid, but many states do provide them. Many states cover bilateral cochlear implants as of the writing of this book, as a result of many appeals that have been undertaken by the Let Them Hear Foundation Insurance Advocacy Program to obtain such coverage. These states include Texas, Massachusetts, Minnesota, Arkansas, Oklahoma, California, New York, and Nebraska.

Medicare has enabled the -50 bilateral modifier for cochlear implant surgery. So, in principle, Medicare has agreed that it will pay for bilateral cochlear implantation. However, it has not established a separate set of criteria for who is eligible to receive the second implant. This is especially important for individuals who have already received one implant and may have good results with it. As of the publication of this book, the authors are not aware of Medicare having covered a sequential bilateral cochlear implant without a long and involved appeals process taking more than sixteen months.

Other Important Health Insurance Concepts

It is extremely important to know whether your health insurance plan is self-insured or traditionally insured. The answer to this question will dictate which laws apply in the event that there is a dispute between you and your insurance company.

The answer to this question hinges entirely upon who bears the risk of loss if the total premiums paid by everyone insured under the plan are not enough to cover all of the claims made under the plan, and correspondingly, who gets to keep the profits if the total premiums paid exceed the total cost of claims paid under the plan.

Larger companies with more than 500 employees, as well as schools and civil organizations, are typically self-insured. In a self-insured plan, the employer is effectively putting money in a pot and paying a company to invest that money and pay claims out of the money in the pot as the claims arise. Companies do this because they believe that it allows them to get the same benefits for their employees for a lower cost than a traditional insurance plan. In these cases, the employer is the true insurer. The insurance company listed on your insurance card is merely a third-party claims administrator, processing claims based on rules defined by the insurer/employer. The federal law known as ERISA only applies to these insurance plans.

All individual health insurance plans, and most plans through smaller employers, are traditionally insured. The law of the state where the insurance company is established governs any disputes. For example, if you work in Oregon, but your small company is headquartered in Texas, then it may be possible that Texas law applies to your dispute with your insurer, even though you live and work in Oregon.

Insurer Disputes

Insurers profit from attrition, uncontested mistakes, illegal denials, and missed deadlines. Even when you win a dispute with your insurer, all you win is the service; there are no provisions for denial-related penalties or expenses that you incurred in getting your denial overturned, short of court-ordered punitive damages, which are extremely rare.

Appeals

When an insurer denies a service you have requested, or refuses to pay a claim after you have received the service, you start the dispute process with internal appeals. There is always at least one level of appeal internal to the insurer, and generally (but not always) a second level of appeal.

If you have exhausted all of your internal appeals, you must then look at appeals levels that are available external to the insurer. Some insurers have a voluntary review panel or external review process, people with traditional insurance frequently have state independent medical review options, and some people with self-insured plans have ERISA arbitration or review committees within their employers that may be available to them. Regardless of whether the plan is traditionally insured or self-insured, if the denial is discriminatory and the insurance is through employment, the individual may be able to file an Equal Employment Opportunity Commission

(EEOC) or ADA complaint against the employer.

Refusal to Preauthorize

The appeals process is only available to those individuals who have actually received denials to requests for either preauthorization (if you have not yet received the service) or a claim (if you have received the service). If the insurer issues a letter saying that it is merely refusing to preauthorize—that is, it won't say yes or no before you receive the service—that is not a denial, and the appeals process is not available to you. Some insurers, for example, never preauthorize in-network surgeries that do not require an overnight hospital stay. If you have one of these insurance plans, and the insurer later determines the procedure was not medically necessary, it will refuse to pay and you will likely be on the hook for the entire cost unless you can win the appeal.

A refusal to preauthorize is not the same as an outright denial. When an insurer refuses to preauthorize a treatment, piece of equipment, or service, what it is saying is, "We won't look at this until after you do it. If we find it is medically necessary, we'll pay for it, but we won't make that determination until after you receive the service."

While just about any insurance company can refuse to preauthorize, the two insurers that are best known for this tactic are Medicare and Blue Cross/Blue Shield for federal employees. Medicare has its own appeals process, and you may not use the insurance commissioner of your state to intervene, which makes the appeals far more difficult and take a much longer time to resolve. Blue Cross Federal-covered members who are federal employees almost never have access to their state insurance commissioners.

Refusal to preauthorize means that all Blue Cross Federal and Medicare appeals are retrospective. Retrospective appeals take much longer to resolve and have a much lower rate of success. To have the best opportunity to get a service covered by an insurer that does not preauthorize, you need at a minimum a letter of medical necessity from your physician and a recent audiogram proving that the level of hearing impairment warrants the service or equipment being requested.

What do you do if you have an insurer that refuses to preauthorize cochlear implant surgery? First and foremost, unless you can write a check for $60,000 without flinching, you need to find a flexible provider and facility. If an appeal is required, it could be nine months or even longer from the time of surgery until the facility gets paid. Keep in mind that the insurer may not be obligated to cover complications caused by a surgical procedure that it refuses to provide approval for. Secondly, you should negotiate a cash rate and payment plan in advance of the surgery should you not win your appeal.

Be aware that a statute of limitations applies to all denials. If you miss any of the appeal deadlines, you lose your right to continue your appeal. Therefore, you need to start your appeal process as soon as possible after you receive either the explanation of benefits (EOB) showing a zero amount being paid, or a "notice of adverse determination." The appeal deadlines for each level vary from state to state. For example, in Oklahoma, the deadline to file a second-level appeal is two weeks, whereas in Florida the law states that you have one year. This is why it is very important to know which state's law governs your appeal, and keep track of those deadlines!

Prospective vs. Retrospective Appeals

Although the appeals process is generally identical, the timelines and outcomes are very different depending on whether the appeal is prospective (which means you have not yet received the service) or retrospective (which means you have received the service).

First, retrospective appeals take an average of twelve to eighteen months from the date of the initial denial to resolve, depending on your region. During this time, your provider, facility, anesthesiologist, etc., will want to be paid. Prospective appeals can average thirty to sixty days in the quicker states and six to nine months in the longer states.

Second, retrospective appeals on a nationwide basis have a much lower chance of success than pre-service appeals. Across all insurance denials in the United States, 80 percent of pre-service denials are eventually overturned, while only 36 percent of retrospective appeals result in overturning the denial. The argument is no longer about whether your medical condition is going to be treated; the argument is about who is obligated to pay for it.

Types of Health Insurance Denials

Health insurers are required by law to state the reason for denial at the time they deny service. The most common reasons for denials for treatment related to hearing impairment include:

- The service/equipment being requested is not medically necessary.
- The service/equipment is being requested by an out-of-network service provider that is not covered under the health insurance contract.
- The service/equipment being requested is excluded under the health insurance contract.
- The service/equipment being requested is experimental or investigational.
- The service/equipment being requested is for a preexisting condition.

How to Structure Your Appeal

Every successful appeal of a health insurance denial is about making it more expensive for the insurer to continue to say "no" than to say "yes." The information in your appeal should be specifically targeted to the reason the health insurer has issued the denial.

Denials Based on Medical Necessity

In these cases, the insurer is arguing that the procedure being requested is not medically necessary, so the argument needs to focus on why it is. Objective test results are the key component to overturning these types of denials. Appeal arguments should also include the psychological and long-term impact, and the cost to the insurer, of the treatment not being received.

Denials Based on an Out-of-Network Service Provider

Insurance companies are obligated to provide you with a competent medical provider, not the best medical provider. However, if the in-network service providers are not competent to provide you with the medical treatment that you need, the insurer must approve your treatment with an out-of-network service provider at in-network rates. In order to prevail in these types of appeals, you must visit the proposed provider to determine his or her qualifications, and then target your argument to why that provider is not qualified and yours is.

Denials Based on Contract Exclusions

It is the position of the Let Them Hear Foundation Insurance Advocacy Program that blanket exclusions for cochlear implants or implantable hearing devices in employer-provided group insurance are illegal under both the EEOC and the ADA. This applies regardless of whether the company is self-insured.

Denials Based on the Treatment Being Experimental/Investigational

If your insurer argues that a treatment is experimental or investigational, you will need to demonstrate that it is not. If your insurer has cited research papers to show that the procedure is experimental or investigational, you should review those papers for both timeliness and audience. In addition, your arguments should focus on the following:

- Research papers supporting the procedure

- The need for speech recognition in noise

- The need for sound localization

- Safety

- Other medical conditions

If your insurer is denying a cochlear implant for a child under twelve months old because it is considered experimental or investigational for this age group, you can also focus on the following additional arguments:

- Special case

- Not approved by FDA, so "off-label"

You will typically face a four-month appeals process, so begin the authorization process by six months, and as a backup plan, schedule two surgery dates, with one scheduled after the first birthday.

Denials Based on Hearing Aid Exclusions

In 2006, a Federal Circuit Court of Appeals determined that health insurance plans that contain exclusions of coverage for hearing aids do not provide a legitimate basis for the insurer refusing to cover cochlear implants. The same court also found that ambiguities in health insurance plans should be read in favor of the patient. In addition to this case, there are several hundred online references from widely varying groups stating that cochlear implants are not hearing aids.

More recently, the newer version of the Americans with Disabilities Act (the Amendments of 2008, which took effect January 1, 2009) specifically updated **the definition of "disability,"** stating **that mitigating measures** such as **aides or accommodations** had **no bearing in determining whether a disability qualifies under the law**. This removed any argument that once a person had a cochlear implant or hearing aid, their hearing impairment no longer qualified them as disabled. Because of this new language, the largest insurer in the United States, UnitedHealthcare, started offering hearing aid coverage in most of its health insurance plans.

Denials Based on Preexisting Condition

As discussed above, your chances of getting these denials overturned differ greatly depending on whether you have an individual plan or a group plan. Exclusions for preexisting conditions in group plans are always temporary, lasting no more than eighteen months from the first date of insurance. Preexisting condition exclusions in individual plans can be permanent.

Foundations/Charities

There are some foundations that can help offset the financial costs of treatment for hearing impairment. These foundations can be especially beneficial to those people stuck "in between"—making too much money to qualify for government insurance, but not enough to afford treatment using their own financial resources.

Several organizations have well-known and long-established programs focusing on assisting individuals with hearing impairment in obtaining hearing aids, cochlear implants, and related services.

Audient, an Alliance for Accessible Hearing Care

http://www.audientalliance.org/

The Audient program, an affiliate of the Northwest Lions Foundation for Sight & Hearing (NLFSH), is designed to assist individuals with hearing impairment who have low incomes. Qualified participants are required to pay a low cost for products and services. Providers in the Audient Alliance network agree to provide comprehensive hearing health care. Audient income-qualifies the participants and manages the database of outcome measures. The Lions Club also sponsors a second program, the Affordable Hearing Aid project. You can find information on this program at:

http://lionsclub.org/EN.our-work/health-programs/hearing-programs/index.php

The Hearing-Impaired Kids Endowment (HIKE) Fund, Supported by Job's Daughters International

http://www.thehikefund.org/

The HIKE fund has given away more than $3 million in hearing devices in the past twenty years. It serves individuals with hearing impairments up to age twenty, and the children can reapply for new devices every four years.

The Starkey Hearing Foundation

http://starkeyhearingfoundation.org

Starkey Corporation, a major U.S.-based manufacturer of hearing aids, began a foundation almost thirty years ago with the mission to deliver hearing aids to individuals who could not afford to buy them. Currently, the Starkey Hearing Foundation delivers 20,000 hearing aids annually through more than 100 hearing missions a year in countries stretching from the United States to Vietnam.

The Gift of Hearing Foundation

http://www.giftofhearingfoundation.org/

The Gift of Hearing Foundation is dedicated to increasing access to and awareness of cochlear implant surgery. The foundation will also keep abreast of and support areas of research as well as legislation that can impact both the cost and awareness factors.

Cochlear Implant Awareness Foundation (CIAF)

http://www.ciafonline.org

CIAF provides information, resources, and support to persons who may be eligible for this life-changing technology. Its founder, Michelle Tjelmeland, and her daughter are both bilateral cochlear implant users.

Colorado Neurological Institute (CNI) Cochlear Implant Assistance Fund

http://www.thecni.org/utility/showArticle/?objectID=974

Through a cooperative effort of Cochlear Americas, Advanced Bionics, and Med-El, as well as a team of dedicated medical professionals, this program is able to assist qualified candidates needing cochlear implants. Device costs and some other fees are waived, and the total cost to the patient ranges from $10,000 to $20,000, well below the $120,000 cash-pay price charged by many institutions to individuals without insurance coverage.

Other Funding Sources

Other possible funding sources, depending on your region and age, can include:

- Area agencies on aging

- Centers for independent living

- Union benefits

- Veterans Administration

- Vocational rehabilitation

- Service clubs, including business and professional women's clubs, Civitan International, Kiwanis International, Pilot International, Quota International, Rotary International, Sertoma International, and Shriner's International

Clinical Trial Participation

Every time a device manufacturer comes out with a new piece of hardware or software, it must go through a clinical trial to establish its safety and effectiveness before the United States Food and Drug Administration will approve its sale to the general public. Generally, individuals who participate in these clinical trials receive the device and related services for free in exchange for the commitment to complete all the appointments necessary for the manufacturer to compile the data on the person's use of the device.

The government must approve clinical trials. A database containing a list of clinical trials and whether or not they are accepting new applications (i.e. "enrolling") is located at http://www.clinicaltrials.gov.

Key Takeaways

1. Treatment for hearing impairment-related issues and assistive listening devices can be extremely expensive.

2. There are several different types of health insurance options out there. It is important to understand your options and what restrictions, if any, may apply.

3. If you are employed, see if your employer has an FSA account you can set up and then pay for the hearing aids with pre-tax dollars.

4. Look into private health care financing options. There are zero interest financing options dedicated to health care costs, such as Care Credit and Chase Health Advance.

5. All states have government funded Medicaid programs for children aged twenty-one and younger.

6. You have the right to appeal if an insurer denies a service you may have requested.

7. The appeal should be structured in a way that targets the reason the insurer has issued the denial.

8. There are several foundations that can help offset the financial costs of treatment.

9. An individual who participates in a clinical trial generally can receive the device and related services for free.

10. Everyone should look at http://www.betterhearing.org/pdfs/e-Guides/Financial_Assistance_for_Hearing_Aids.pdf. Many of the entries in this

book are very location-specific—for example, only for residents of a particular county in Kentucky—but it is a very large guide, and some may work for you.

Chapter 7

Hearing Impairment and the U.S. Public Education System

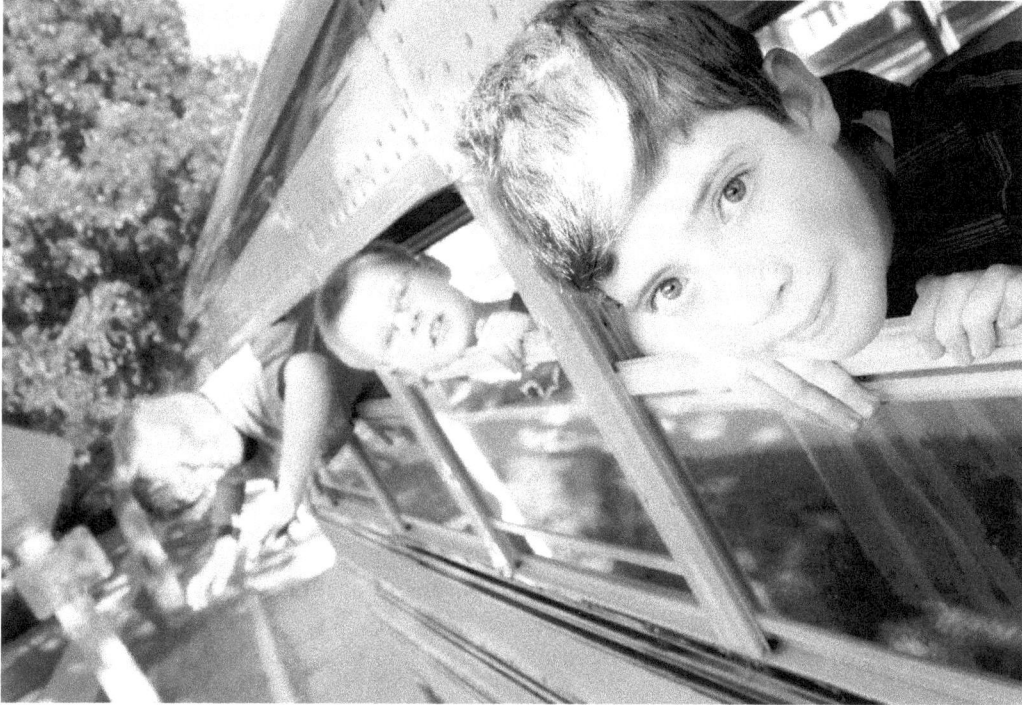

Introduction

This chapter is intended to introduce you to some very high-level concepts regarding what services might be available to you through the public school system, how to determine which law applies, and some of the magic language to use when requesting these services. This chapter is not intended to be a comprehensive, detailed evaluation of how to get the services you are entitled to from the public school system for a child with a hearing impairment. The federal law that governs this, the Individuals with Disabilities Education Act (IDEA), alone is 1,600 pages long, and there are entire books and entire careers dedicated to this one narrow area of law.

IDEA

IDEA stands for the Individuals with Disabilities Education Act. It is a federal law that was initially enacted in 1975, and has been overhauled and reenacted twice: once in 1997, and most recently in 2004. Though IDEA was reenacted in 2004, the corresponding federal regulations implementing IDEA 2004 did not take effect until October of 2006.

Hearing impairment and deafness are specifically listed disabilities within IDEA, as long as the hearing impairment is of a sufficient level that it affects the child's educational performance. There are no specific decibel loss requirements necessary to meet the criteria. Some children may find that their educational performance is impaired with a bilateral mild loss, while for others, a unilateral moderate-to-severe loss may not be sufficiently large to impair their education.

Children with any disability listed in IDEA, including hearing impairment, are entitled to a Free Appropriate Public Education (FAPE) that is specially designed to meet their unique needs. Furthermore, IDEA requires that children with disabilities must be placed in the Least

Restrictive Environment, which is an educational setting that does not impose unnecessary restrictions on either the child or the family with respect to location, nor does it force the child to use a communications modality other than the one the family has selected.

This is important because only a few decades ago, many children with significant hearing impairments were diverted to residential schools for the deaf as their only educational options. Residential schools for the deaf are now rarely considered the Least Restrictive Environment for educating a child with a hearing impairment, unless the family wants a signing program and the school district is incapable of providing one.

Educational environments that may be offered to you under IDEA include mainstream general education, special classes in a mainstream school setting, special schools, home instruction, and instruction in hospitals and other residential institutions.

IDEA Misconceptions

There are many misconceptions, both among school districts and among families, about what IDEA can and can't do for a child with an educationally significant disability.

Common District Misconceptions in Implementing IDEA

While the IEP team has broad discretion and flexibility in creating the IEP based on the needs of the child, unfortunately, the fact is that IDEA is an unfunded mandate. Federal law requires that all states provide these services to children, but the federal government funds less than 21 percent of the total costs. Therefore, public school districts frequently, though illegally, plead poverty in attempting to avoid their obligations under IDEA, even though they are forbidden from doing so under federal law.

It is important for every parent to understand that under IDEA, the district is not allowed to make presumptive denials—in other words, it cannot deny services without doing an assessment. Some examples of presumptive denials would include the parent of a hearing-impaired child being told any of the following by a school principal:

- When requesting information about available Total Communication programs, being informed that "the district does not support Total Communication."

- When requesting an FM system for their child, being informed that "we only do sound-field systems."

- When requesting use of the FM system during private therapy sessions, being informed, "FM systems can only be used on school grounds."

- When requesting an assessment for purposes of evaluating whether there is a need for an IEP, being informed that a child must be failing in school to qualify for services.

Each of these cases constitutes a presumptive denial because the parent is being denied the request out of hand, without the district having made even the most basic investigation into the individualized educational needs of the child. Unfortunately, many district employees do not realize their obligations under IDEA and make these types of illegal statements on a regular basis, because it is the way things have been done in the past. It is your job as the parent to understand what your rights and the district's obligations are under federal law, and to make your requests in such a way that the district knows you are educated on the topic of what your child is entitled to.

Common Parental Misconceptions About Their Rights Under IDEA

While IDEA guarantees equal opportunity for all children regardless of any educationally significant disabilities they may have, it does not guarantee a specific level of achievement or even a regular high school diploma. Parents should never confuse the Free Appropriate Public Education all children are entitled to with being able to request what is "best" for their child, or even what they prefer for their child. Parental convenience is not a factor in determining whether a child is receiving FAPE, and parents are not entitled to the "Cadillac" of educations at 100 percent public expense.

Section 504

Children who have disabilities, but whose disabilities do not interfere with their ability to progress in a regular general education setting, are not eligible for special education services under IDEA, but are entitled to a 504 Accommodation Plan.

504 plans are appropriate for children who have hearing impairments that are not considered educationally significant. A common example of this might be a child with a single-sided hearing impairment who only requires an FM system in order to function in a normal classroom setting, or a child who wears hearing aids and only requires speech therapy, as opposed to program-based accommodations.

The major differences between an IEP and a 504 plan are:

- 504 plans are governed by civil rights law (ADA).

- IEPs are governed by education law (IDEA).

- IEPs contain greater provisions than 504s for:
    - Progress reporting
    - Discipline protections

- "Stay put" when the child changes schools and the new school does not agree with the plan put in place by the old school

Early Intervention/Individualized Family Service Plans (IFSPs)

As discussed in the chapter on infant hearing screening, the primary concept behind early intervention is that the earlier treatment begins for children with hearing impairments, the more successful the outcome. Twenty years ago, before universal infant hearing screening, children were frequently not identified with hearing impairments until they had significant language delays, and just before they were ready to start preschool. Today, many children with hearing impairments are identified before they even leave the newborn nursery, giving their families the opportunity to begin treatment before the children have speech and language delays. Addressing the issue before language delays occur creates a better and less expensive outcome for everyone, including the government.

"Early intervention" is also a catchall phrase for a federally mandated program that is implemented in every state in an attempt to identify children from ages zero to three years who have disabilities that are likely to be educationally significant when they begin kindergarten. The concept behind early intervention is that if these children receive services and therapy for their educationally significant disabilities starting at an extremely young age, they are likely to require fewer services over their lifetimes and be more successful in the educational setting, and have more overall potential as adults.

Every state has an early intervention program, but not every state calls its program "early intervention." Those that do use this term often abbreviate it as EI. Another common name is

First Steps.

Early intervention is implemented using a document called an Individualized Family Service Plan (IFSP). One or more meetings are held between parents or guardians and early intervention personnel to develop the IFSP. Significant features of IFSPs include:

1. IFSPs are only for children under the age of four years.

2. IFSP services are provided through Part C of IDEA.

3. IFSPs name a service coordinator to help the family during the development, implementation, and evaluation of the IFSP.

4. IFSPs are centered on the family, whereas IEPs are based upon a formal education setting, such as a school. Frequently, services identified in the IFSP are provided in the child's home.

5. IFSPs include outcomes targeted for the family. For example, if the family and early intervention staff agree that the child's mode of communications will include signing, then the IFSP can include the provision of sign language instruction to the family, in addition to the child.

6. IFSPs include the concept of "natural environments." Therefore, IFSP activities can take place in the home or on a playground, whereas IEP activities almost universally take place at the school or in a therapist's office.

7. IFSPs include activities undertaken with multiple agencies beyond the scope of Part C. These are included to integrate all services into one plan.

For each child receiving services under an IFSP program, prior to age four, a transition meeting must be held to reassess the child's need for services and implement the services that continue to be required under an IEP rather than an IFSP.

Individualized Education Programs (IEPs)

IEP stands for Individualized Education Program. An IEP is a combination of:

• A meeting

• A document

• A description of a child's entire educational program

An IEP must include current educational status, goals and objectives, instructional setting or placement, and related services and assistive technology required to provide the child the Free Appropriate Public Education in the Least Restrictive Environment that he or she is legally entitled to under IDEA.

The child's needs dictate what placement, services, and technology are included in an IEP. Assessments done either by the school district, the family, or both determine the baseline of the child's current educational level, reasonable goals and needs, and a plan for how to get the child to where he or she should be at the end of the period of time that the IEP covers.

Children in Private Schools

A school district's obligation to provide services can even extend to children who are homeschooled or unilaterally placed in a private school setting by the parents.

Child Find is a component of IDEA that requires states to identify, locate, and evaluate all children with educationally significant disabilities, from birth to age twenty-one, who are in need of early intervention or special education services.

Under no circumstances is a school district allowed to provide services in a parochial school setting. However, the school district may offer to provide speech therapy, audiology, or other related services at the public school that the child would be attending if he or she were not attending the parochial school in its place. The district may also offer to provide assistive technology that can be used in the parochial school setting. The same is true for homeschooled students.

The reason that services cannot be provided within the physical parochial school setting is that the provision of government-paid employees in a religious school setting is viewed as a violation of the First Amendment to the U.S. Constitution, which guarantees a separation of church and state. However, failing to provide these children with any support whatsoever is shortsighted. There is no guarantee that a child who is currently in a parochial school setting will stay in that setting for his or her entire thirteen years of public education. A child with a hearing impairment who receives no support is more likely to fail the parochial setting and return to the public education setting, where he or she will be playing a catch-up game that is hard to win. Therefore, the compromise is that some districts, within the constraints described here, offer limited services to these children, but only in school district or neutral settings.

A Supreme Court case (NYC Board of Education v. Tom F.) came to the conclusion that parents do not have to try a public school setting and fail in that setting in order to receive services in a private school at which they have chosen to enroll their child.

Important IEP Development Concepts

There can be no disputing that every child is different, and children with hearing impairments are no exception. Even children with largely identical audiograms will have different strengths and weaknesses and acquire information differently, which affects the services that they require in the educational setting and who is best suited to deliver those services. Furthermore, 40 percent of children with hearing impairment have some other educationally significant need that must be addressed in addition to their hearing impairment. Therefore, it is extremely important to remember, and sometimes remind the school district, that the "I" in IEP stands for "Individualized."

The role of the parents in developing the IEP cannot be underestimated. Parents are frequently their children's best advocates. Under IDEA law, parents always need to be offered the role of a full IEP team member. The overall process for developing an IEP generally adheres to the following timeline:

1. Either the parent or a professional determines that a child requires special education services.

2. When the parents make this determination, they write a letter to the appropriate special education administrative office requesting that an IEP meeting be held.

3. Within some fixed period of time from the receipt of the request for an initial IEP, the school district must provide the parents with an assessment plan and a copy of a notice of parent rights. In California, under Cal. Ed. Code 56321(a), this period of time is fifteen days.

4. The parents must determine whether they will consent to the assessments proposed by the school district within a specified number of days of receipt of the assessment plan. In California, under Cal. Ed. Code 56321(c), this period of time is also fifteen days.

5. The assessment must be completed and the IEP developed within a fixed number of days of receiving the written consent. In California, under Cal. Ed.

Code 56344, this period of time is fifty calendar days. Generally, the number of days does not include official school vacations or holidays.

6. Once the assessment is completed and before the IEP is developed, the school district must provide proper notice to the child's parents of the date the IEP meeting will take place. The notice must include the purpose, time and location of the meeting, who will attend, and a notification of the parents' ability to invite others to the IEP who have knowledge or special expertise about the child. Because it is presumed that the parents will participate in the IEP process unless they intentionally opt out, it is typical for the school district to informally contact the family by phone to agree to a meeting date, location, and time before the notice is officially sent out to all parties who will attend the meeting. This also allows the family to specify which professionals, if any, they would like to attend the IEP meeting.

7. Many states require that upon request, parents be allowed to examine and receive copies of all school records within a fixed number of calendar days from the date the request was made in writing or verbally. In California, under Cal. Ed. Code 56504, this period of time is five calendar days.

If the parent requests an IEP meeting without the need for new assessments, slightly different timelines generally apply. This might occur when a child already has a valid IEP in place, and only an amendment is being requested, or the request is purely for technology based on existing assessments and no new assessments are required. In California, under Cal. Ed. Code 56343.5, the IEP must be held within thirty days (not including days in July or August) from the date of receipt of the written request.

IEP Life Cycle

There is a definitive life cycle to IEP development. Frequently, it takes the better part of a school year to completely develop and implement an IEP. Therefore, starting early is essential. Providers of services to school-aged children with hearing impairments frequently refer to April as "IEP month" because it is the time of the year that they are most busy writing recommendations for FM systems, speech therapy, and acoustical classroom modifications.

A typical IEP development life cycle is as follows:

Phase I   Collecting relevant information (fall)

Phase II   Assessment of current information and program and tailoring of current or future IEP goals (winter)

Phase III   Preparation and meeting to finalize IEP content (spring)

Phase IV   Resolving disputes (spring/summer)

Phase V   School begins

Phase VI   Progress reporting

IEP participants typically include the following, with asterisks indicating those whose attendance is mandatory:

• Speech pathologist

• Audiologist

• Special education teacher (at least one) *

- Special education administrator*

- Parents*

- Child (six years or older)

- Outside experts/support persons

- Mainstream teacher (at least one) *

- Medical personnel (as needed)

- Psychologist

- Language interpreter

IEP Assessment Plans

The district must provide the parents with a copy of the assessment plan prior to testing. The parent should review the assessment plan to make sure that it addresses the following issues:

1. Are all areas of concern being addressed?

2. Are the tests appropriate for the age and ability level of the student?

3. Are test percentage outcomes properly normed?

4. Is the examiner qualified and experienced?

5. Will testing be done over an appropriate number of sessions?

6. Will the tests be performed in an appropriate setting?

7. Are all tests valid based on previous testing?

8. In the case of triennial evaluations or psychological tests, does the psychologist have experience working with hearing-impaired students?

Assessment Tools for Children with Hearing Impairments

Any test being used to assess the abilities of a child for the purposes of an IEP evaluation must:

- Not be discriminatory on a racial or cultural basis

- Be given in your child's native language or other mode of communication, unless it is clearly not feasible to do so

- Measure a disability and not limited English language skills

Common assessment tools used to evaluate the speech and language of children with hearing impairments up to age three include:

- The Battelle Developmental Inventory
- Receptive Expressive Emergent Language Scale (REEL 2)
- Infant Toddler Meaningful Auditory Integration Scale (ITMAIS)
- Cottage Acquisition Scales for Listening Language and Speech (CASLLS)
- Preschool Language Inventory
- Expressive and Receptive One Word Peabody Picture Vocabulary Tests
- Spontaneous Language Sample

Common assessment tools used to evaluate the speech and language of children with hearing impairments from age four through twelve include:

- Preschool Language Inventory
- Cottage Acquisition Scales for Listening Language and Speech (CASLLS)
- Listening Test
- Word R Test
- Spontaneous Language Sample
- Peabody Picture Vocabulary Test Receptive and Expressive
- Wechsler Individual Achievement Test Boehm Test of Basic Concepts
- Boehm Test of Applications
- Durrell Listening Comprehension Test

- Ling Speech Evaluation
- Phonological Awareness Test
- Test of Problem Solving (TOPS)

Independent Education Evaluations

Generally, district personnel do initial assessments. However, if there are no district personnel qualified to do the assessment, or you do not agree with the assessment results, you may request that the district conduct an independent educational evaluation (IEE), which is performed by qualified professionals who are not district employees.

Prior to requesting an IEE, the following steps must occur:

• You agree in writing to allow district staff to assess your child.

• The assessment is performed.

• The results of the assessment(s) are reported to you.

• You disagree with the results.

In response to your request for an IEE, the district must take one of two actions:

• Provide the IEE at public expense, or

• Initiate a due process hearing to demonstrate that the district's evaluation was appropriate

In the first situation, if the school district agrees to provide an IEE at no cost to you, it may do so in a variety of ways. It may give you names of individuals who are qualified to assess, suggest a state-supported agency (such as a diagnostic school), or even arrange to have an employee of another school district do the evaluation. In any case, certain conditions, qualifications of evaluators, and standards spelled out in IDEA must be met. If the district agrees to provide an IEE at public expense, it doesn't necessarily mean it will pay for an assessment by the professional of your choice.

If the second outcome occurs, the district will request a due process hearing to ask an independent adjudicator to agree that the assessment it performed followed appropriate IDEA standards for evaluation and was conducted by qualified individuals. After hearing testimony from both the district and the parents and reviewing pertinent records, the due process adjudicator (sometimes referred to as a "hearing officer") has an option of either accepting the district's assessment, or ordering an independent evaluation.

Of course, parents always have the option of obtaining an independent evaluation at their own expense. The district is always obligated to consider the results of such an assessment at an IEP meeting. However, giving consideration to the report doesn't mean the district has to agree with the results or accept the recommendations made by the professional who did the assessment. If the district does use new information from the IEE you paid for which was not part of its assessment to develop goals for your child's IEP, the district may be responsible for reimbursing you for a part or all of the cost you incurred to have the evaluation performed.

IEP Disputes

If the parents and the school district cannot reach full agreement on all components of the IEP and the IEP is not signed, either the parent or the local education agency may request a due process hearing from the Special Education Hearing Office (SEHO). The SEHO has forty-five days from the day it receives the due process hearing to make a decision. This is true in all states, as federal law codified at 34 C.F.R. Sec. 300.511 governs it. Due process (sometimes also referred to as a "fair hearing") is an expensive and time-consuming process. Most states have either optional or mandatory pre-hearing mediation, which may allow for faster resolution of the dispute. Generally these meetings are confidential, meaning that anything discussed or offered by either the parents or the district cannot be introduced into evidence at the fair hearing at a later time. Another important aspect of pre-hearing mediation is that neither side is allowed to have attorneys present.

Credentialing

The rules pertaining to special education teacher credentialing changed with IDEA 2004 to bring the rules in line with No Child Left Behind. Any public elementary or secondary school special education teacher must have full state certification in special education or must have passed the state special education licensing exam *and* hold a license to teach as a special education teacher. However, the rules are different for charter schools, which only have to meet the requirements set forth in their particular charter laws. For charter schools, minimum emergency credentials are not allowed, and the teacher must hold at least a bachelor's degree.

IEP Meeting Preparation

The two keys to a successful IEP meeting are organization and information gathering. Parents who have all their information supporting their requests in writing in advance of the IEP meeting are far more likely to get the outcome they desire. Parents can prepare for IEP meetings by:

1. Carefully reviewing all documentation provided by the district, including the notice, the assessment plan, assessment results, and progress reports from previous IEPs if they exist

2. Bringing in outside parties or objective evidence, such as grades, to document the child's current status

3. Drafting sample goals, rather than coming into the meeting with a blank sheet of paper

4. Mentally prioritizing new goals and requests

The definition of a compromise is that neither party gets exactly what they want, but each party can live with the results. Frequently this is what happens with IEPs. Parents never get as much as they want, and schools frequently have to do more than they want. However, given the tedious nature of due process hearings, and the risk of the losing party bearing the costs for both parties, it is rare for either the family or the school district to be so unhappy with what the other party is prepared to settle for that they are willing to introduce either the significant delay or the financial risk involved with proceeding to court.

IEP Goals

IEP goals must be appropriate, definable, measurable, and reviewed and assessed on a regular basis. IEPs must contain both short-term and long-term goals. Long-term annual goals identify the anticipated achievement to be made during the school year, including the method for evaluating progress. Short-term goals list multiple milestones necessary to achieve annual goals, generally in sequence.

Each and every IEP goal should contain:

1. A baseline defining the child's current level of mastery of the goal topic

2. An anticipated date of completion of the goal

3. The method for determining whether the goal has been met

4. The person responsible for reporting on goal progress

5. Goal progress reporting dates

IEP Goals Specific to Hearing Impairment

There are many IEP goal areas that are common to children with hearing impairment. These include goals for articulation, receptive and expressive language, and academic goals specifically tailored to either the issues created by the hearing impairment, or some other educationally significant issue that the child is concurrently experiencing. Goals can also address equipment. Examples of some of these goal topics include the following.

Articulation Goals

- Oral motor skills

- Specific phoneme development

- Speech prosody, such as intensity, pitch, and duration

- Structured setting vs. spontaneous setting

Receptive Language Goals

- Detecting and identifying Ling sounds

- Closed set versus open set word recognition

- Detection versus discrimination

- Understanding speech in the presence of competing noise

- Following directions

- Auditory memory

- Answering question forms

- Listening to stories and gathering information

Expressive Language Goals

- Babble

- Vocabulary

- Single words to word combinations

- Express needs

- Relate events

- Carry on give-and-take conversation

- Use grammatically correct language

Academic Goals

- Phonics

- Vocabulary (general and subject-specific)

- Idioms, pronouns, tense

- Concrete and abstract comprehension

- Spelling

- Simple sentences, not necessarily grammatically correct

- Grammatically correct sentences

- Paragraph and story writing

- Word problems

General Behavioral Goals

- Respond appropriately in give-and-take conversation

- Initiate play with other children

- Child learns to advocate for him/herself

- Hearing aid, implant and FM system use

- Appropriate classroom placement

- Participates in classroom conversation

- Looks at other students when they are talking

- Child organizes schoolwork

Equipment Usage Goals

- Child will report when batteries are dead

- Child will initiate usage of FM system

- Audiologist will check FM system function every thirty days

IEP Goals Not Specific to Hearing Impairment

It is extremely important for all parents to understand that in the public education system in the United States, there should be no such thing as an informal testing accommodation. All testing accommodations, even those as simple as the provision of written directions as opposed to verbal instructions, need to be documented in writing in the child's IEP. This is for two crucial reasons. First, it ensures that the school consistently implements a child's accommodations from classroom to classroom, rather than depending on what one teacher feels like doing for a given assignment or test in a particular class. Second, standardized testing services outside school districts, such as the Educational Testing Service, who is in charge of SAT testing, require proof of necessity of testing accommodations before they will grant accommodations within their testing programs.

As a result, it may be necessary for your child to have IEP goals pertaining to educational areas where accommodations are necessary for him or her to receive a Free Appropriate Public Education because of the impact that hearing impairment has on his or her education. Goals can also be established for other related areas of education, including adaptations in how children are tested, requirements for their assignments, how instructions are provided, what types of assistance children can receive in the classroom, and how children are graded.

Some common types of accommodations in these areas can include testing adaptations, assignment adaptations, changes to grading, and modifications to classroom or subject matter presentation.

Testing Adaptations

- Change essays to multiple choice

- Reduce number of multiple-choice answers

- No true or false questions

- No essay questions

- Provide a word bank (very important for general education classes)

- Matching in groups of five

- Fill-ins in groups of five

- Accept short answers

- Open book or open notes

- Allow students to record or dictate answers

- Reduce spelling list for spelling tests

- Do not penalize spelling or grammatical errors, except on tests specifically covering those areas

- Extend time frame or shorten length of test

- No Scantron answer sheets

- Provide written instructions to student

- Read test to student

- Allow student to replay verbal sections of tests as many times as necessary (good for foreign language classes for older students)

- Provide study guide prior to test

- Allow student to do test on a typewriter or computer

- Have more tests covering smaller units of test material

- Highlight key directions

- Take test in alternative site, such as a quiet room

- Allow use of calculator

Assignment Accommodations

- Uncluttered worksheets

- Give all directions both in writing and verbally

- Write assignments on the board

- Do not penalize for spelling or grammatical errors, except on assignments specific to those topics

- Show samples including visual models

- Reduce assignments

- Read written work to student

- Allow student to submit all assignments on computer rather than handwrite

- Provide alternate assignment/strategy when demands of class conflict with student capabilities

- Avoid penalizing for poor penmanship

- Allow parental assistance with homework

- Communicate homework expectations with parents, including sending home a homework notebook that must be signed and returned by parents

- Check for student's lesson comprehension

- Shorten tasks to accomplish longer tasks

- Allow student to work with a buddy on assignments

- Assign the student a note taker whose notes can be used in completing assignments

Classroom/Subject Matter Presentation Accommodations

- Read text aloud

- Provide written text for all verbally presented material (song lyrics for choir, for example)

- Small group instruction

- Provide an accurate copy of notes or key points written on the board or overhead

- Utilize manipulatives, such as blocks, to teach math concepts

- Highlight critical information

- Pre-teach necessary subject-specific vocabulary and concepts

- Do not call on to read aloud in class

- Check student's lesson comprehension

- Provide written study guides

- Assign a "study buddy"

Grading Accommodations

- Use pass/fail

- Use a modified scale

- Credit for partial completion

- Consider effort in assigning grade

- Credit for participation

- Copy of tests to special education teacher

- Copy of all tests to parents

- Teacher will notify special education teacher when grades drop below C-

Miscellaneous Accommodations

- Avoid timed activities or provide extended time

- Preferential seating

- Cues for staying on task

- Provide a quiet place to work

- Opportunity for physical movement

- Seat next to a good role model

- Daily check-in with special education teacher

Bad IEP Goals and Good IEP Goals

Bad goal: He will imitate modeled lip and tongue placements.

Why this is a bad goal: "Imitate" does not imply accuracy; there is no measurement.

Good goal: He will be able to achieve a developmentally appropriate range of tongue and lip movements 75 percent of the time as measured by his speech therapist.

Bad goal: She will develop fifty new words (nouns and verbs).

Why this is a bad goal: "Develop" is too vague; there is no distribution and no measurement. Alternatively to providing a list of words to learn, for younger children, a baseline vocabulary can be attached.

Good goal: She will appropriately articulate and use thirty-five new nouns and fifteen new verbs as measured by an end-of-semester assessment by her Teacher of the Deaf (TOD) using the vocabulary list attached at Appendix A.

Bad goal (for a toddler):   He will categorize like items and label the grouping.

Why this is a bad goal: This goal is inappropriate for a child who is just beginning to talk. It is important that the goals be age-appropriate. Future goals can be written into IFSPs that cover those ages, such as, "At age 3 ½, ..."

Good goal: None in this area

Bad goal: She will follow simple directions using ten common verbs.

Why this is a bad goal: There is no measurement, no definition of the term "simple," and no list of verbs to choose from.

Good goal: She will follow eight one-step directions, which will include syntactic structures such as possessive-entity and entity-location, as measured by the classroom teacher using any of the verbs listed in the PBK words list attached in Appendix A.

Logistics Associated with Delivery of IEP Goals

Once the basic IEP goals are agreed on between you and the school district, a significant number of logistical issues remain that must be addressed regarding how the services necessary to achieve those goals will be delivered. Some of these issues include:

- Is each service individual and/or small group?

- How often is each service going to be delivered?

- Who is the responsible person for each portion of the service?

- How is progress toward the goals to be reported?

To address these logistical issues, it is absolutely essential to establish a structure for communication between professionals working with your child. Measurement toward goals, and plans for reevaluating services if goals are not met, are also crucial to any child successfully reaching his or her IEP goals. If this is a trial placement and there is concern about whether the environment is the best fit for the child, then a short-term, two-month progress report and a follow-up IEP meeting should be scheduled as part of the initial IEP implementation plan.

For children being placed in a mainstream environment who are in kindergarten or later grades, the government requires that as part of the IEP, the percentage of time the child is learning in a mainstream environment be listed in the IEP document. To avoid future IEP meetings where decisions are made based on teachers' undocumented feelings about how a child is doing, something which can rarely be challenged by parents who are in the classroom infrequently, it is important to identify how the mainstreaming experience will be monitored: an aide in the classroom, a teacher or outside therapist visiting on a regular basis, etc. It is important that this data be collected in a notebook and reviewed over time so that summary conclusions without individual data points supporting them are not relied upon when determining what services the child needs to continue his or her successes going forward.

The school district is obligated to either provide, or reimburse the parent for, transportation expenses if the services agreed to are not available in the child's home school. These obligations are covered by IDEA regulations Section 300.24 (b)(15), 300.456, and Appendix A Question 33. Transportation arrangements should be specifically outlined in the IEP to avoid confusion later. Parents can use transportation as a negotiating chip. For example, if a district has the option of providing services at two locations and the parents prefer one location over another, they can offer to waive their right to transportation reimbursement to make the district more amenable to agreeing to the services at the location the parent desires.

If a child is at risk of having skills regress during the summer vacation period, IEPs can address the need for an extended school year program (i.e. summer school), which would allow the child to continue services during vacation periods.

Assistive Technology

As discussed in the introductory section of this chapter, presumptive denials of any kind, including requests for assistive technology, are not allowed under IDEA. Therefore, requests for assistive technology, such as personal FM systems specific to a child's hearing devices that are recommended by outside service providers, must be considered by the district. The district is always entitled to refuse the request if its own providers have done an independent assessment and do not agree with the outside opinion you have provided, but it is obligated to provide explicit and supporting reasoning behind why it disagrees with your experts. These grounds are essential in order for you to take the next step and appeal the denial to an independent mediator or a due process hearing officer if you so desire.

If your district does grant the request for assistive technology, just getting the equipment is not enough. There are several other peripheral issues that should be addressed in the IEP in addition to the actual provision of the assistive technology:

1. Are there equipment usage goals?

2. Who needs to be trained to use the equipment?

3. If the student's regular teacher is absent, who is charged with training the substitute teacher? Planned absences may be handled differently than emergency absences.

4. How often will the equipment be checked, and who will check it, to ensure that it is functioning properly?

5. If the equipment is misplaced or out for repair, what is the backup plan?

6. Can the student use the technology in learning settings outside of the school site?

On the above list, item 6 is clearly the most contentious, and school districts are frequently quite reluctant to allow equipment to leave their control. However, the key legal issue that parents need to focus on is whether FM system use outside the classroom is necessary for a child to receive FAPE, which it almost always is. Homework, outside therapy sessions, field trips, and tutoring outside of school grounds are all activities where it can easily be argued that it is necessary for a child to use the assistive technology in order to receive FAPE. Therefore, it is unreasonable, and probably legally unsupportable, for a district to issue a blanket refusal against allowing the FM system to leave the school. However, it is reasonable for the school district to require the parents to be liable for damage or loss to the FM system when it is in the parents' control outside the school. Therefore, it is even more crucial that insurance be maintained on shared equipment.

Related Services

IDEA lists "related services" that are to be provided by the school district when needed; these include "transportation and such developmental, corrective, and other supportive services as are required to assist a child with a disability to benefit from special education." IDEA identifies a long list of services, which includes audiological and speech services, but then further states that this long list of services is not exhaustive and may include other developmental, corrective, or support services "as may be required to assist a child with a disability to benefit from special education."

Audiology Services

Audiologists who screen, assess, and identify children with hearing impairment generally provide audiology services. In the educational context, audiologists:

1. Determine the range, nature, and degree of the hearing impairment

2. Make recommendations for other professional involvement for the habilitation of hearing

3. Provide language habilitation, auditory training, speech reading (lip reading), speech conservation, and other programs

4. Determine the child's need for a hearing device, select and fit the hearing device, and evaluate the effectiveness of the amplification

Many school systems, in particular smaller districts, do not have the diagnostic facilities necessary or even an audiologist on staff. Some districts may contract with facilities to provide these services directly; others find it easier to reimburse parents for the cost associated with seeing the child's private audiologist.

Before IDEA 2004, which took effect in October 2006, a court case concluded that related audiological services included mapping and cochlear implant programming sessions. Congress was concerned that this court case opened the door to districts being required to pay for cochlear implant surgery itself, so it modified both Part B and Part C of IDEA to specifically exclude maintenance of surgically implanted medical devices. The new language states: "Related services do not include a medical device that is surgically implanted, the optimization of device functioning, maintenance of the device, or the replacement of that device."

Speech-Language Pathology Services

Speech-language pathologists (SLPs) address the needs of students with communication disabilities, regardless of whether a hearing impairment is present. In the context of the educational setting, SLPs:

1. Screen, identify, assess, and diagnose disorders of fluency, language, articulation, voice, and oral-pharyngeal function, and cognitive/communication disorders

2. Provide speech and language services for the habilitation or prevention of communication disorders, including augmentative and alternative communication systems

3. Make recommendations for other professional involvement for the habilitation of speech or language disorders

Interpreters and Aides

Interpreters and aides can be assigned on a child-specific basis, if necessary to achieve

FAPE in the Least Restrictive Environment. Because of their expense, districts are reluctant to provide these services unless they are proven to be absolutely necessary. As the parent is solely in charge of the child's choice of communications modality, the interpreter can be of any kind, with the most common being ASL, SEE, and Cued Speech. An oral interpreter—someone who repeats what is being said, but facilitates speech reading—is also possible.

Children with multiple disabilities may require aides throughout their education process. Children who are adapting to devices may require aides temporarily and then no longer need them. As they get older, children with hearing impairment, no matter how well they have adapted to their situations, may discover that as they take classes with more difficult vocabulary or classes that require significant note taking, they once again require the assistance of an aide.

Acoustic Assessments

Bad classroom acoustics have an adverse effect on all children, but the effect is more apparent for children with hearing impairment. One of the most common complaints among people who wear hearing aids is that *everything* is amplified, because even the best devices can only make limited distinctions between speech and background noise. Individuals wearing hearing devices often have difficulty comprehending conversations in noisy environments, because the words are competing with all the other background noise in the room. In audiology, this competition is referred to as the signal-to-noise ratio, where the signal is the speech and the noise is all non-speech sounds. Acoustical assessment is the process by which rooms are analyzed for background noise. Sometimes very simple modifications can be made to create a quieter classroom environment that results in more important sounds, like voices, being heard more clearly.

If the background noise is so chronically bad that it creates an environment where a child with a hearing impairment cannot possibly receive the Free Appropriate Public Education that all children are entitled to, then the district is obligated to solve the problem: either by moving the child (and possibly the entire class) into a more suitable classroom, or by making acoustic modifications to the classroom to restore the balance so the child can receive FAPE.

In order to make classroom modifications, parents need to start very early, up to a year before the child will actually be in the classroom. It helps if the family is familiar with the terms and standards recommended by the American Speech-Language-Hearing Association (ASHA) with respect to unoccupied classroom acoustics:

1. Background noise levels should not exceed 30 dBA or Noise Criteria NC-20 curve.
2. The signal-to-noise ratios should be greater than 20 decibels.
3. Reverberation times should not exceed 0.4 seconds.

You need to be specific about which physical areas need to be assessed. These could include the classroom, the therapy area, or an auditorium. Auditoriums are incredibly difficult to address and may be better and more cheaply handled by using FM systems, rather than attempting to reduce the background noise when several hundred students are simultaneously present.

Create an Acoustic Inventory

To get an idea of just how bad classroom background noise can be, leave a tape recorder running in an occupied classroom at the seat your child will be occupying for a couple of hours. When you play the tape back, you will likely hear a reverberant mess of sound. If there were any voices recorded during this experiment, they may be hard to understand because of the background noise.

Creating an acoustic inventory is the first step to solving the problem. First, go through the classroom with a critical ear and make an inventory of all the things that generate sound. This could be any kind of machine with a motor that is constantly running, such as air conditioners, furnaces, fans, and doors that are constantly being opened and closed. Write everything down so that you can review the list later and figure out ways to quiet these everyday noises.

Next, look for—or listen for—surfaces that cause noise through contact. These could be hardwood or tile floors, chairs that make scraping sounds when they move, doors that make noise when opened or closed, or things banging on desks.

Finally, listen to see if there are areas of the classroom that promote the echoing of sounds. Step into the middle of the room and clap your hands. Do you hear something immediately afterward? Try making a short, loud sound with your voice. You will be able to tell if the room has acoustics that are too lively.

Appliances

Now you have your acoustic inventory. For each of the items we've discussed, there are generally methods that can be used to make them quieter. Motors can sometimes be made quieter through the use of soft rubber pads or filters, which absorb the vibrations that would otherwise be transmitted to the floor and heard as noise.

Many electrical devices cause unnecessary sound because they are not secured properly and are vibrating against something. Ceiling fans are a good example of this. If the fan is a little bit loose, it can make an irritating sound at certain speeds. Make sure all devices like this are securely attached.

Proper installation can also cut down on noise from window air conditioners. Test all the screws that hold the air conditioner in place and tighten them if necessary. Running the air conditioner on the lowest setting will make it less noisy. This also applies to fans.

Surfaces

For floors, the obvious thing is to use carpets. This really helps to cut down on general ambient noise as well. Carpets are not convenient in all areas; linoleum flooring will always be quieter than harder flooring such as cement, hardwood, or tile. In areas where the flooring cannot be modified, a few small area rugs will help cut down the noise level.

One of the largest sources of noise in any classroom is the scraping of desk and chair legs against the floor as students get up and down several times per day. An easy way to eliminate this is to attach tennis balls to the legs. Cut a large X in a tennis ball with a utility knife large enough for the leg to fit through, but small enough so that it will stay on when the table or chair is lifted. Pads that are nailed to the bottom of the leg serve a similar purpose and can be bought in hardware stores. For classrooms that have large quantities of chairs, ask your local sports club to collect and donate "dead" tennis balls—they may have lost their bounce for playing good tennis, but they will still eliminate noise from chairs, and the low or free price will satisfy cost-conscious district managers.

For tabletops where group projects are done, tablecloths or placemats will absorb the sound of whatever activity is being performed on a hard surface. Doorframes can be padded so that the door doesn't slam when it is closed. Weather stripping material, which can be acquired at almost any hardware store, is perfect for this. Small rubber stoppers mounted on the door, combined with a small wall-mounted pad, can substantially reduce the sound of the door hitting the wall when it is opened.

Ambient Room Noise

For lively sounding rooms, carpeting on the floor can help absorb noise and reduce echoing. Full-length curtains or wall hangings will make it even quieter. Any hard surface is going to reflect sound, but when it is covered with cloth, the sound will be absorbed. Tablecloths or mats can be used on tables. Windows can be covered with sheer curtains. Walls can be covered with acoustic tiling, which will also reduce the amount of sound echoing throughout the room.

Recent IEP Legal Cases

There has been a great deal of recent interest by the Supreme Court in cases regarding children's rights under IDEA. There were only five cases in the first thirty years after IDEA was enacted. There have been four cases in the past two years. Unfortunately, some of the more important cases have been decided in favor of the districts.

For example, under the ruling in *Schaffer v. Weast*, it is now the rule in the entire nation that the party contesting the student's placement or services has the burden of proof in establishing that the other party's decision is incorrect. Since 98 percent or more of the time it is the parents contesting the district's denial of services or placement, the parent almost always has the burden of proof in these matters.

However, no Supreme Court decision has ever supported the proposal that the school district can ever choose the communications modality to be used in teaching the child. Cases and documentation prior to the implementation of IDEA 2004 which support the parent's right to choose the child's communication modality include:

"It is especially important that a full continuum of alternative placements is made available to meet the unique communications and related needs of deaf and hard-of-hearing students."

OSEP Letter to Cohen, 25 IDELR 516 (1996)

"An oral-aural approach to teaching a child with a cochlear implant is not a methodology issue, but rather what the child needs to satisfy the goal of talking."

W.F. v. Flossmoor School Dist. 161, 38 IDELR 50 (IL 2002)

In *Eureka Union School Dist.* 28 IDELR 513 (SEA CA 1998), the parents of a child with a cochlear implant were reimbursed for the cost of a private oral program because the district program was heavily weighted toward ASL, which would have required the child to learn a new form of communication.

In *San Mateo-Foster City School Dist.* 28 IDELR 527 (SEA CA 1998), a three-year-old who had been in AVT therapy since she was two months old, with siblings who also used AVT, required an AVT placement to receive FAPE and also satisfy California education law, specifically 56000.5(b) and 56441.2.

In *D.D. vs. Foothill SELPA,* OAH No L-2002020373, the court found that a school that provided personnel with the requisite minimum credentials was not sufficient; a proven track record of working with children with cochlear implants was essential in order for the child with a hearing impairment to receive FAPE.

Key Takeaways

1. Know whether you want an IEP or a 504. They each have different protections and different requirements, and 504 plans do not allow requests for things that

modify academic programs.

2. Specify the qualifications for the personnel you are requesting. Not a "paraprofessional," but a "paraprofessional with three years of experience working with learning-disabled children." Not a "sign language interpreter," but an "ASL interpreter with an NIC certification for K-12 education."

3. Come to the meeting prepared with an outside recommendation for the equipment you want your child to use to achieve FAPE, complete down to the brand name and model number. Schools always want to use the equipment they have previously purchased, because it is less expensive for them, but it isn't always best for your child. If you come with an outside recommendation, typically from your child's audiologist, the district has to consider it as part of the process and find a reason to rebut it.

4. When you come to an agreement with the school about assistive technology, don't stop just at the equipment. Consider everything that goes with the equipment, including: What do you do as a backup if the equipment is being repaired? Who pays for the batteries for the equipment? Who trains the substitute teacher in how to use the equipment in the case of a planned absence? In the case of an emergency absence? Does the equipment go offsite for fieldtrips? Can you take the equipment home over vacations?

5. Mondays are terrible days to schedule speech therapy, AVT, or audiology rehab sessions. There are too many holidays on Mondays, and IEPs usually do not allow make-up sessions for sessions that are missed on regularly scheduled school holidays.

6. Remember that IEPs have seasons, and plan your appointments accordingly. IEPs for the fall generally start in April. Nothing ever happens over the summer.

7. If you do not agree with the results of the school district's Independent Education Evaluation (IEE), you are entitled to a second one with people that you select at district expense, unless the district first goes through due process and proves to a hearing officer that the second IEE is unnecessary.

8. Don't forget about test fatigue. Children who are tested and retested with the same tests will get false results. Make sure you agree with the district about what tests are being used.

9. Make sure the IEP includes a plan for tracking progress and compliance in between reporting periods. Many people use a notebook that is sent back and forth between the teachers and parents to discuss what the child is doing and any issues he or she may have related to hearing impairment and IEP/504 goals.

10. Have a plan in advance for what you will do if your child's educators go out of compliance with the IEP/504 plan. How will you report it? Who will you report it to?

Chapter 8

The Future of Treatment for Hearing Impairment

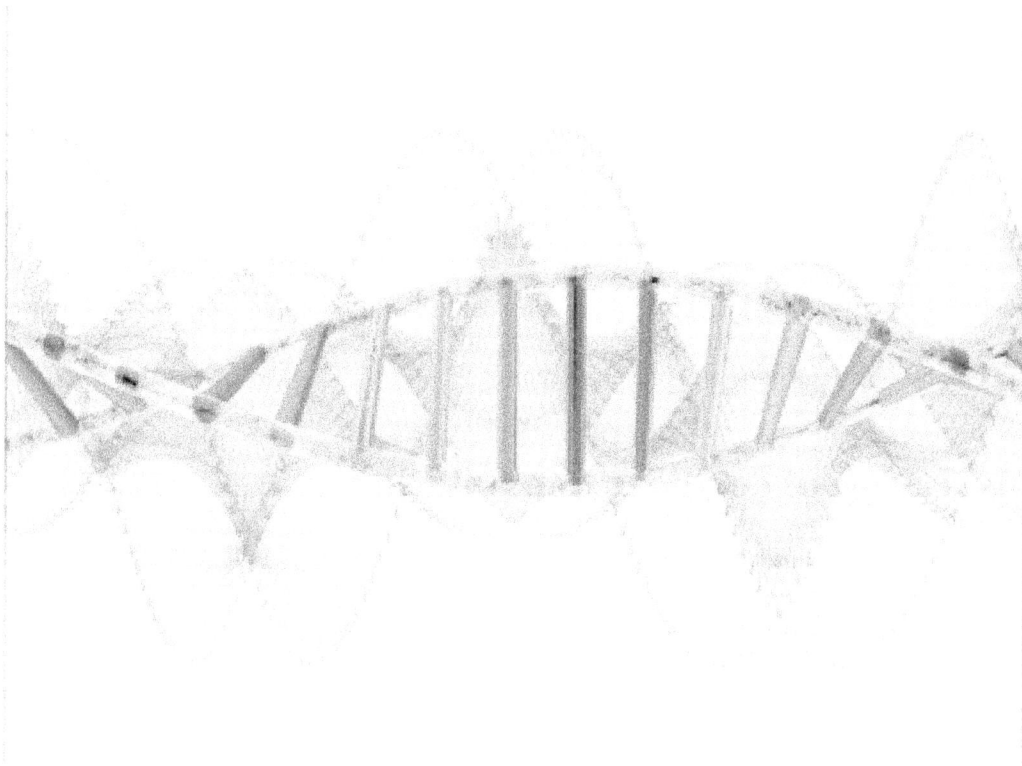

Hybrid Cochlear Implants

Remarkably, the human ear can make sense of a combination of mechanical hearing and the electrical hearing of a cochlear implant in the same ear. In some patients, a small, shorter-than-normal electrode from a cochlear implant can be inserted without damaging what hearing remains in the operated ear. The remaining hearing can be stimulated with a hearing aid, again wearing both devices in the same ear. Early clinical trials show improved hearing in noise and more natural sound perception and music perception.

Reduced Age of Cochlear Implantation

Since their inception roughly twenty years ago, cochlear implants have been used in younger and younger patients. Data is absolutely clear that younger is better in terms of learning and outcome. Expect this to continue to ages well below twelve months, the current FDA-approved age. With informed consent by parents, many children have received cochlear implants at less than one year of age. The youngest in our clinical experience is bilateral devices at five months of age. We expect the FDA-approved age of implantation to drop in the near future. Discussion with your hearing health care providers will help you determine the best age of cochlear implantation for your child and whether one or two are needed.

Completely Implantable Cochlear Implants

Companies are at work on technology to allow all components of a cochlear implant to be placed under the skin. This presents a number of challenges, including making the device small enough to be practical and to work with children. Another major issue is battery life. This is a bigger challenge for cochlear implants than for pacemakers because a cochlear implant, which runs multiple electrodes in "always on" mode, has much greater power needs. The ability to recharge an implanted battery will be a must. Also, as anyone who owns a camcorder knows, batteries have only so many charge/recharge cycles before they cease to hold a charge. This means revision surgery may be needed to change the power supply.

Microphones have recently become adequate to pick up sound well when placed under the skin. This requires a thin tissue layer over the microphone, and some surgeons are concerned about the safety of such an arrangement in the long term. While this solution is appealing from a cosmetic standpoint, few parents or patients would be willing to trade better looks for worse function.

Until some of these and other technical considerations are addressed effectively, these theoretically interesting devices will not enter mainstream clinical practice. Nonetheless, we predict such offerings will be options for future patients and will find their place in the treatment of hearing impairment, first in adults and then in children.

Hair Cell Regeneration Research

Hair cells are essential for hearing and balance. Without them, we would be completely deaf and constantly disoriented. If hair cells are damaged in any way, we suffer permanent hearing impairment or balance degeneration. New research, however, is showing that there may be a way to regenerate damaged hair cells.

Hair cells got their name because under a microscope, they look as though they have a tiny hair protruding from them. These hair-like structures are called stereocilia, and they bend in response to sound. There are two types of hair cells: auditory and vestibular. Auditory hair cells are located in the cochlea of the inner ear, and are responsible for detecting sounds. Movements of the hairs are translated into electrical signals, which are transmitted to the brain and interpreted as sound.

Vestibular hair cells are responsible for our sense of balance. These are located in a different part of the inner ear: the vestibular organs. While damaged auditory hair cells can be compensated for with the use of hearing aids or replaced through cochlear implantation, there is no replacement or cure for damaged vestibular hair cells.

Hair cells do not function in isolation, but need to be connected to the auditory centers of the brain through nerve fibers. The challenge of hair cell regeneration, therefore, is not only to replace damaged hair cells, but also to somehow get them to reconnect to the nerves so they can send information to the brain.

Sounds that are louder than 90 decibels will cause temporary damage to human hair cells. The hair cells become flattened, resulting in short-term hearing impairment. Usually, they will regain their shape in a short time. Long-term exposure to loud sounds, however, will result in permanent hearing impairment. Other things that can damage hair cells include ototoxic drugs (drugs which cause hearing impairment), disease, and aging.

Once human hair cells have died, they cannot be regenerated. In other species, however, hair cells are constantly regenerated. Researchers are now working to see if this process can be somehow applied to human hair cells, thereby restoring lost hearing.

Hair Cells in Birds

In the mid-1980s, scientists discovered that adult birds can regenerate hair cells. In researching this phenomenon, it was discovered that birds have the ability to recover their hearing when loud noises or drugs have damaged the hair cells. The recovered hearing seems to be equivalent to the hearing ability the bird had before the damage occurred.

In addition to birds, amphibians such as frogs can also regenerate hair cells. Mammals, however, do not have this ability. Researchers are trying to discover the mechanism behind amphibian and bird hair cell regeneration and see if it can be applied to humans.

There seem to be two major factors in this process: the regeneration of the hair cell and the reconnection of the hair cell to the nerve cells. It appears that when hair cells are produced, they secrete molecules called trophic factors, which attract nerve fibers. When the hair cells are connected to the nerve cells, hearing is restored.

The major obstacle in duplicating this process in humans is the difficulty of generating new hair cells. This has to be done through a process of cell division. Recent experiments using guinea pigs, mice, and rats have succeeded in promoting cell division within the inner ear using growth-promoting molecules. So far, similar molecules for human use have not been found, but at least the possibility of hair cell regeneration in mammals has been confirmed.

Transplants and Gene Therapy

Another approach that is being investigated is to transplant hair cell precursors into the inner ear. Precursors are cells from which other cells are formed. Unfortunately, hair cell precursors have not yet been identified, but embryonic research is being done to identify which cells in the embryo develop into hair cells.

Gene therapy is also being researched as a way to stimulate hair cell growth. Already, the genes responsible for stimulating precursor cells into hair cells have been identified. This method for regenerating hair cells within humans is being actively investigated, with steady progress.

Hair Cell Regeneration—The Treatment of the Future

At this time, nothing can be done to replace hair cells in humans. Damaged hair cells must be compensated for with the use of hearing aids or circumvented by the use of cochlear implants. There is no currently no therapy for damaged vestibular (balance) hair cells.

Research over the past twenty years, however, has shown amazing potential. Scientists are making frequent breakthroughs in understanding the mechanisms involved in hair cell regeneration and its possible application to human hearing impairment. Once the specific molecules involved in hair cell regeneration have been identified, it may become a viable treatment. However, most hair cell regeneration scientists and otology experts believe that this is likely at least fifteen years in the future.

About the Authors

Joseph B. Roberson, Jr., M.D., is the CEO and managing partner of the California Ear Institute, president of the Let Them Hear Foundation, and the medical director of the Adult and Pediatric Cochlear Implant Program at Children's Hospital Oakland. Dr. Roberson is an internationally renowned specialist in otology, neurotology, and skull base surgery and is board certified in otolaryngology. Dr. Roberson is a member of the American Neurotology Society and the AAO-HNS. He serves as a consultant for several leading manufacturers of equipment for hearing impairment, including Cochlear Corporation, Advanced Bionics Corporation, Medtronics-Xomed, NeuroPace, and SoundID. He is widely published in peer-reviewed medical journals and textbooks and regularly presents to physicians, audiologists, and the general public in many different venues and locations. Additionally, Dr. Roberson is a faculty member and former chief of otology-neurotology-skull base surgery at Stanford University.

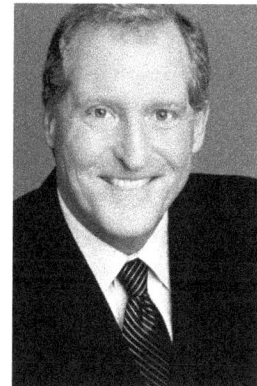

Sheri Byrne-Haber, B.Sc., J.D., is the director of advocacy for the Let Them Hear Foundation. Ms. Byrne-Haber founded the LTHF insurance advocacy program in 2004 specifically to assist individuals who are hearing-impaired and their families in obtaining services they have been denied by health insurers. In addition to this program, Ms. Byrne-Haber has been very active in the hearing-impaired community for the past decade, working with parents of newly diagnosed children with hearing impairments in their quest to gather information on treatment options, education options, and insurance reimbursement for their children's conditions. Ms. Byrne is a former attorney who also has a degree in computer science and has three daughters, one of whom is severely hearing-impaired.

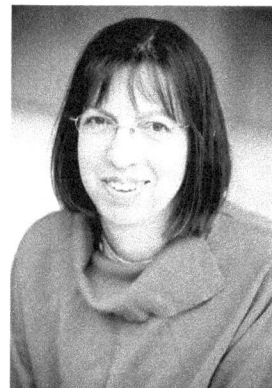

Caitlin Roberson has worked in corporate and nonprofit settings, leveraging her hands-on experience for aligning message with market in the B2B and B2C sectors. Her efforts tripled a national beauty site's social media following from 12,000 to over 36,000 in six months. As associate director for a medical nonprofit, she exceeded annual projections by developing relationships with media outlets nationwide. Examples include CBS, *Time Magazine,* and *The Washington Post.* Caitlin also helped Napa Valley wine producers promote their unique value propositions to high-income-bracket collectors in a philanthropic environment. Her efforts brought the miracle of hearing to hearing-impaired children in third-world countries. Caitlin's work has received university and state recognition. Her work has appeared in magazines, blogs, and e-books nationwide. She completed her B.A. in English after three years at UCLA, *magna cum laude.*

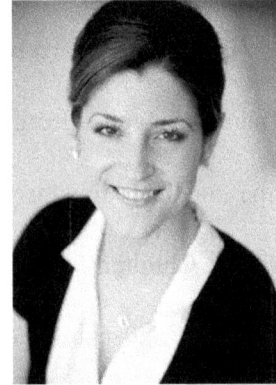

Definitions

Causes of Hearing Impairment

Acquired	Nongenetic and noncongenital causes of hearing impairment such as meningitis, infection, chemotherapy, head injury, or age
Auditory neuropathy	Disorder in which sound does not get transmitted normally from the cochlea to the auditory nerve
BOR	Branchiootorenal syndrome, sometimes referred to as Melnick-Fraser syndrome
CHARGE Association	Coloboma [eye], heart anomaly, atresia [choanal], retardation [mental and growth], genital anomaly, ear anomaly
CMV	Congenital cytomegalovirus; occurs when the mother is infected with the cytomegalovirus during pregnancy
Congenital	Hearing impairment present from birth
Connexin	Connexin 26 and 30 mutations are recessive genetic errors and are the most common sources of congenital profound hearing impairment.
HFM	Hemifacial microsomia, commonly associated with conductive loss due to congenital aural atresia and microtia

Meniere's disease	Typically causes unilateral hearing impairment, always accompanied by vestibular imbalance
Meningitis	Can cause mild to profound hearing impairment, frequently accompanied by vestibular imbalance
OAV	Oculo-auriculo-vertebral spectrum (can include hemifacial microsomia, Goldenhar syndrome)
Otosclerosis	Arthritis in the middle ear bones, typically in people aged fifty and up
Ototoxic	Drugs that cause hearing impairment; gentamycin and chemotherapy are the most common. Vicodin in large doses is also known to be ototoxic.
Prematurity	Responsible for a significant number of cases of hearing impairment due to associations with high bilirubin, ototoxic drug exposure, CMV, auditory neuropathy, or some underlying genetic cause that triggered the premature birth.
Progressive	A hearing impairment that gets worse over time
TCS	Treacher-Collins syndrome: a genetic, craniofacial birth defect that is characterized by a range of distinctive facial anomalies.
Usher's syndrome	A recessive genetic disorder associated with progressive sensorineural hearing impairment and retinitis

pigmentosa, which leads to both deafness and blindness

Viral infection	Can cause unilateral or bilateral hearing impairment overnight
Waardenburg syndrome	Hereditary hearing impairment associated with blue eyes and white streaks in the hair

Tumors Associated with Hearing Impairment

Acoustic neuroma	Tumor of the acoustic nerve; removal frequently results in hearing impairment
Cholesteatoma	Benign cyst of the internal auditory canal; can result in significant conductive hearing impairment
Glomus tumor	Tumors of the arterial portion of the glomus body; surgery frequently results in sealed-off ear canal and significant conductive hearing impairment
NFM II	Neurofibromatosis Type II; causes acoustic neuromas on both acoustic nerves

Types of Hearing Impairment

Conductive	Cochlea functions correctly, but something is blocking the sound from getting to the cochlea

Mixed	Loss is part conductive, part sensorineural
Sensorineural	Nerve-based hearing impairment; the sound is getting to the cochlea but is not being properly processed

Ear Deformities

Aural atresia	Missing ear canal
Canal stenosis	Incomplete atresia, narrow ear canal
Microtia	Missing or deformed outer ear
Stapes fixation	Congenital malformation or fusion of the stapes (one of the three bones of the middle ear)

Tests Associated with Hearing Impairment

ABR	Auditory brainstem response (same as BAER)
Audiogram	Hearing test
BAER	Brainstem auditory evoked response (same as ABR)

CT scan	Computerized tomography scan
HINT	Hearing in noise test
IHS	Infant hearing screening
MRI	Magnetic resonance imaging
Tympanogram	Test of pressure on eardrum

Terms Associated with Balance Disorders

BPPV	Benign paroxysmal positional vertigo, a disorder caused by problems in the inner ear
CDP	Computerized dynamic posturography
Dix-Hallpike	Diagnostic maneuver used to diagnose BPPV
Nystagmus	Involuntary eye movement

Audiogram Terms

AC	Air conduction
BC	Bone conduction

CNT	Could not test
Cookie bite	A loss that is exclusively (or worse) in the middle speech frequencies, with the high and low frequencies relatively spared; the audiogram picture looks like a cookie with a bite taken out of it, hence the term
dB	Decibel, a measure of sound level relative to hearing (logarithmic)
DNT	Did not test
Hz	Hertz, a measurement of the frequency of the sound being tested
kHz	Kilohertz, or 1,000 hertz
Mild hearing impairment	21 to 40 dB in children, 26 to 40 dB in adults
Moderate hearing impairment	41 to 55 dB
Moderately severe hearing impairment	56 to 70 dB
Normal hearing	Anything under 20 dB in children, 25 dB in adults

Profound hearing impairment	91 dB or higher
PTA	Pure tone average, the average decibel level of the three speech frequencies where the person reliably responds to tones (500, 1,000, 2,000 Hz)
Severe hearing impairment	71 to 90 dB
SNHL	Sensorineural hearing impairment
Speech banana	A banana-shaped range of frequencies and decibel ranges where the majority of English speech occurs, between 1 kHz and 4 kHz
SRT	Speech reception threshold
WNL	Within normal limits

Hearing Devices

BCHA	Bone conduction hearing aid
Bi-CI	Bilateral cochlear implant
CI	Cochlear implant

FM system	A piece of assistive technology that uses FM radio signals to send sound from the person wearing a microphone directly to hearing-impaired individuals
HA	Hearing aid
Sound-field system	Like an FM system, but uses "boom box" or speakers mounted in the room rather than headphones or hearing aids on the receiver side

Surgeries

Atresia repair	Creation of an ear canal
Auricular reconstruction	Repair of deformed outer ear; can be done utilizing one of two methods: rib graft or Medpor (plastic)
PORP	Partial ossicular replacement prosthesis
Stapedectomy	Removal of stapes bone
TORP	Total ossicular replacement prosthesis
Tympanostomy	Ear tubes, sometimes called pressure equalization (PE) tubes
Tympanoplasty	Surgery on or replacement of the eardrum

Communications Choices

ASL — American Sign Language

Auditory-oral — Speech-based communication

AVT — Auditory-verbal therapy

Speech reading — Formerly known as lip reading

TC — Total Communication

Hearing Professionals

ENT — Ear, nose, and throat doctor

Audiologist — In the United States, the individual who programs hearing aids and/or cochlear implants and performs hearing tests

Otolaryngologist — Another name for an ENT

Otologist — ENT who focuses exclusively on ears. In the United States, a board-certified otologist has an additional two years of training after the general four years of ENT training is completed.

SLP   Speech-language pathologist

TOD   Teacher of the deaf

Hearing Impairment Abbreviations

DHH   Deaf/hard of hearing

HI   Hearing impaired

HOH   Hard of hearing

SSD   Single-sided deafness

Insurance Terms

COBRA   Consolidated Omnibus Budget Reconciliation Act of 1985, the law in the United States that allows you to retain your insurance for a short time (generally eighteen months) after you leave a job

DME   Durable medical equipment

EOB   Explanation of benefits

EPO	Exclusive provider organization
ERISA	Employee Retirement Income Security Act, the federal law that governs self-insured plans
HIPAA	Health Insurance Portability and Accountability Act, the federal law that governs the requirement to maintain the privacy of one's medical data. HIPAA also guarantees that you can convert your group insurance plan to an individual plan when you leave a job or your COBRA extension runs out.
HMO	Health maintenance organization
HSA	Health savings account
INP	In-network provider
OONP	Out-of-network provider
OOP	Out of pocket
POS	Point-of-service insurance plan
PPO	Preferred provider organization
TPA	Third party administrator

School System

FAPE	Free Appropriate Public Education
IEP	Individualized Education Program
IFSP	Individualized Family Service Plan (the equivalent of an IEP for children under three)
LRE	Least Restrictive Environment
504 Plan	Spells out the non-academic program changes (modifications and accommodations) that will be needed for students with hearing impairment, which have been determined to not adversely impact their academic performance, to have an opportunity to perform at the same level as their peers

Hearing Aids

Analog	Hearing aids without digital speech processing capabilities
BTE	Behind the ear
Digital	Hearing aids with digital speech processing capabilities

Digitally programmable	Hearing aids without digital speech processing that have programming features that analog aids don't have
Feedback	A high-pitched squeal that occurs when the source of the sound is too close to the microphone. Can be reduced or eliminated with the use of feedback cancellation software, which is frequently a feature of digital hearing aids.
ITC	In the canal
ITE	In the ear

Web Sites

Assistive Listening Devices

Phonic Ear

http://www.phonicear.com/

Listen Technologies Corporation

http://www.listentech.com/

NADY Systems, Inc.

http://www.nady.com/

Sennheiser Electronic Corporation

http://www.sennheiserusa.com/home

Williams Sound

http://www.williamssound.com/

Ear Infections

Otitis media

http://www.medinfo.co.uk/conditions/otitismedia.html

Glue ear

Hearing Aid Manufacturers

ReSound

http://www.gnresound.com/

Oticon

http://www.oticonusa.com/

Phonak

http://www.phonak.com/us/b2c/en/home.html

Siemens

http://www.medical.siemens.com

Starkey Laboratories

http://www.starkey.com/

Widex

http://www.widex.com/

Cochlear Implant Manufacturers

Advanced Bionics

http://www.advancedbionics.com/us/en/home.html

Cochlear Limited

http://www.cochlearamericas.com/

Med-El

http://www.medel.com/us/index/index/id/1/title/HOME

Medical Associations

American Academy of Otolaryngology

http://www.entnet.org

American Medical Association

http://www.ama-assn.org/

Hair Cell Regeneration

Inner Ear Hair Cell Regeneration

Hearing Dogs

NEADS

http://neads.org/

Hearing Dogs for Deaf People

http://www.hearingdogs.org.uk/

Assistance Dogs International, Inc.

http://www.assistancedogsinternational.org/

International Hearing Dog, Inc.

http://www.ihdi.org

Organizations

AAO-HNS American Academy of Otolaryngology-Head and Neck Surgery

http://entnet.org/

AG Bell   Alexander Graham Bell Society

http://nc.agbell.org

ASHA   American Speech-Language-Hearing Association

http://asha.org/

HLAA   Hearing Loss Association of America (formerly Self Help for the Hard
of Hearing)

http://www.hearingloss.org/

JWPOSD   Jean Weingarten Peninsula Oral School for the Deaf

http://www.deafkidstalk.org/site/

Research Bibliography

Bess, F.H., Tharpe, A.M. "Case History Data on Unilaterally Hearing-Impaired Children." *Ear Hear* (1986): 7(1):14-19.

Culberson, J.L., Gilbert, L.E. "Children with Unilateral Sensorineural Hearing Impairment." *Ear Hear* (1986): 7(1):38-42.

Oyler, R.F., Oyler, A.L., Matkin, N.D. "Unilateral Hearing Impairment: Demographics and Educational Impact." *Lang Speech and Hearing Services in Schools* (1988): 19:201-210.

Ovo, R., Martini, A., Agnoletto, M., et al. "Auditory and Academic Performance of Children with Unilateral Hearing Impairment." *Scandinavian Audiology Supplementum.* (1988): 30:71-74.

Jensen, J.H., Borre, S., Johansen, P.A. "Unilateral Sensorineural Hearing Impairment in Children: Cognitive Abilities with Respect to Right/Left Differences." *Brit J Audiol* (1989): 23:215-220.

Bess, F.H., Tharpe, A.M., Gibler, A.M. "Auditory Performance of Children with Unilateral Hearing Impairment." *Ear Hear* (1986): 7:20-26.

Keller, W.D., Bundy, R.S. "Effects of Unilateral Hearing Impairment upon Educational Achievement." *Child: Care Health Dev* (1980): 6:93-100.

Stein, D. "Psychosocial Characteristics of School-Age Children with Unilateral Hearing Impairments." *J Acad Rehabil Audiol* (1983): 16:12-22.

Dancer, J., Burl, N.T., Waters, S. "Effects of Unilateral Hearing Impairment on Teacher Responses to the SIFTER: Screening Instrument for Targeting Educational Risk." *Am Ann Deaf* (1995): 140:291-294.

McKay, S. "To Aid or Not to Aid: Children with Unilateral Hearing Impairment." *Healthy Hearing: Your Complete Hearing Aids Information Source.* Healthy Hearing.com, 2002. Retrieved May 11, 2007.

Reeve, K., Davis, C., Hind, S. "Mild and Unilateral Hearing Impairments: What the Clinicians Think." Poster presentation at A Sound Foundation Through Early Amplification Conference, Chicago, IL. October 2001.

Brookhauser, P.E., Worthington, D.W., Kelly, W.J. "Unilateral Hearing Impairment in Children." *Laryngoscope* (1991): 101(12, pt 1):1264-1272.

English, K., Church, G. "Unilateral Hearing Impairment in Children. An Update for the 1990s." *Lang Sp Hear Serv Schools* (1999): 30:26-31.

Hartvig, Jensen, J., Borg, S., Johansen, P.A. "Unilateral Sensorineural Loss in Children. Cognitive Abilities with Respect to Right/Left Ear Differences." *Brit J Audiol* (1989): 23(3):215-220.

Spitzer, J.B., Ghossaini, S.N., Wazen, J.J. "Evolving Applications in the Use of Bone-Anchored Hearing Aids." *AJA* (2002): 11(2):96-103.

Wazen, J.J., Spitzer, J., Ghossaini, S.N., et al. "Results of the Bone-Anchored Hearing Aid in Unilateral Hearing Impairment." *Laryngoscope* (2001): 111(6):995-958.

Reeve, K. "Amplification and Family Factors for Children with Mild and Unilateral Hearing Impairment." *National Workshop on Mild and Unilateral Hearing impairment: Workshop Proceedings. Breckenridge, CO: Centers for Disease Control and Prevention.* (2005): 20-21.

Jerger, J., Silman, S., Lew, H.L., Chmiel, R. "Case Studies in Binaural Interference: Converging Evidence from Behavioral and Electrophysiologic measures." *JAAA* (1993): 4:122-131.

Davis, A., Reeve, K., Hind, S., Bamford, J." Children with Mild and Unilateral Impairment." In Seewald, R.C., Gravel, J.S., eds., *A Sound Foundation Through Early Amplification 2001: Proceedings of the Second International Conference, Great Britain.* St. Edmundsbury Press, 2002: 179-186.

Peters, B.R., Litovsky, R., Parkinson, A., Lake, J. "Importance of Age and Postimplantation Experience on Speech Perception Measures in Children with Sequential Bilateral Cochlear Implants." *Otology & Neurotology* (2007): 28:649-657.

Sharma, A., Dorman, M., Spahr, A. "A Sensitive Period for the Development of the Central Auditory System in Children with Cochlear Implants: Implications for Age of Implantation." *Ear & Hearing* (2002): 532-539.

Sharma, A., Dorman, M., Kral, A. "The Influence of a Sensitive Period on Central Auditory Development in Children with Unilateral and Bilateral Cochlear Implants." *Hearing Research* (2005): 203:134-143.

Snik, F.M., Teunissen, B., Cremers, W.R.J. "Speech Recognition in Patients After Successful Surgery for Unilateral Congenital Ear Anomalies." *Laryngoscope* (1994): 204:1029-1034.

Breier, J.I., Hisocock, M., Jahrsdoerfer, J.A., Gray, L. "Ear Advantage in Dichotic Listening After Correction for Early Congenital Hearing Impairment." *Neuropsychologia* (1998): 36(3):209-16.

Index

www.ingramcontent.com/pod-product-compliance
Lightning Source LLC
Chambersburg PA
CBHW081653270326
41933CB00017B/3156